And now, she has a good looking body shape at the age of nearly 50, she is still georgeous!

This means that going on diet with 6 meals a day may work if you can live with such diet. Unfortunately, I can't do that.

I love to eat and I looove to eat.

Almost all of my life as an entertainer, I have to maintain my body, that was why I forced myself to be like most other people by trying various diets that tortured my body and consuming dietary pills that only remove excess water in the body, then my body got fat again... one sentence ... I am tired...but now everything has changed ... I can eat my favorite foods, I exercise energically and I have 8 pack-abs at my age of nearly 40 years old ... with cell age at 28 years old. Yes, I am getting younger by time now... the question is how?

So let me tell you a little story first...

About 5 years ago, I went to Hong Kong to get a martial instructor certificate, I spent nearly a week in a rental car with the driver. Interestingly, after the first 3 days, I just knew that the age of the driver is 70 years with the face and physical body like 40 years ... I thought it was impossible ...
So I asked him how can he achieved that?And he shared me a secret...

A secret that did not make sense in my opinion at that time.

He taught me the secret for 4 consecutive days until I knew that he is a former Shaolin Monk in China.

But after I returned to My Country, this idea just disappeared. I was struggling to my old diet with the same stupidity, I did not want to take the risk to try something new ... until the last three months.

I had to host a TV show and had to open my shirt on the scene ... It stressed me out because my body was not that good.

Monks Diet

"**THIS IS AN ANCIENT CHINESE SECRET** that people forget and don't care...

WESTERN world has made a very money oriented business to gain money from supplements and **FAKE** science and illegal drugs to make people looks good.
yet they demand the people to suffer their life by dieting, and fear from lack of supplements..."

"What gets us into trouble is not what we don't know. It's what we know for sure that just ain't so."

— Mark Twain

LET'S START

If you are reading this article, there are several possibilities that happen to you, the first is that you have unattractive body shape or mostly called it fat or chubby

Or **obesity**...

What it is like to be obese? Believe me, I know how it feels ... I have lived overhalf of my life like that ... being bullied at school ... scared of mirrors and scales ...

Only your parents said that you are great ... actually they lied.

I was born with least desirable body type, endomorph.

This means that my genetics WANT me to be fat, isn't it cool?

And it happened to my brother and sister too... the great thing is:my sister went on a strict diet every day by eating red rice and plain chicken breast for almost 20 years before she was introduced to my MD.

Then, I remembered what I learned from the taxi driver. I analyzed his explanation, looking for logical explanations on internet for 1 month to believe that what he said is true and can be tried. Then, I tried. Here I am with 6-pack abs and getting younger and stronger!

Do you know that diet pills are the best selling drug in the world? Almost everyone has purchased, tried diet pills and failed.

Strangely, there are labels in almost all diet pills saying that "must be followed by exercise and food intake regulation", so what does the diet pill for?

Interestingly, we can see why do most diets fail?
In one study, 311 obese women were recruited to join one of the following popular diet programs:

AtkinsDiet, Zona Diet, Diet LEARN atau Diet Ornish (various kinds of diet).

To begin the study, each woman should follow one of the popular diet programs randomly, and they were asigned to follow the program.

Then, before they went on a diet, each woman has attended a series of 8 courses (each course lasted for one hour) explaining how to follow the assigned diet.

After the courseswere completed, they set out to follow their diet for 1 year.

What was the result?

They lose a lot of weight in the first two months, after that they tended to stop the diet. In the end, eventhough they lose weight, but the result was far from what was expected.

- none of them lose wight of more than 11 pounds in a year ... pathetic!

They concluded that the diet did not work, and they might get the wrong program, they also said that they should follow the other programs (they have not seen that results of other diets were the same).

But in my opinion, this failure is much simpler ...

First, all the diets used in this experiment are unable to accurately measure how many calories a person eats in a day. Second, these results indicate that one reason of failed diet is the compliance to the diet itself. I think that there are easier diets.

In other words, the more complicated the diet is, the more likely it will fail in the long run.

- people are unable to comply to diet for a long period of time.

In fact, some researches support my analysis.

In a study published in International Journal of Obesity entitled "Dietary Compliance and successful weight loss among overweight women":

Guess what did they find?

Only 1 out of 12 people complied the diet for a year and she managed to lose 88 pounds, while the remaining participants did not comply to the diet. This means that 100% of people want to have a great body shape but 90% of them do not want to go on a diet because it is too complicated and boring.

More complicated = low probability of success

easy = high probability of success

Hasn't this happened in all areas?

In my opinion, there are 2 most complicated diet rules, namely:

1. **Calculating caloric intake**
2. **Looking for healthy foods to eat (the foods are not tasty).**

But they are getting lazier after knowing that it takes a long time to reduce weight significantly.

The problem is that we are not Arnold Schwarzenegger(American body builder) and would not be, at least I do not want to, he is an amazing person and I really appreciate him as a friend.

But being that Big isn't my dream.

Let's talk a little about him, Arnold Schwarzeneggeris an incredible person and I am very impressed with him, apart from what other bodybuilders say about him. His healthy lifestyle could be a great inspiration for everyone. He goes on an outstanding and very healthy diet, and performs an extraordinary exercise...

But not everyone is Ade Ray, not everyone will survive in the long-run diet as applied by him such as eating red rice or plain breast chicken and various kinds of supplements every day, at least I cannot do that.

I will only be able to eat what he eats for 1 or 2 weeks. I am sorry, I am not that perfect.. GOD! I LOVE FOOD! maybe not a healthy one, but I LOVE TASTY FOOD! just like you all.

Ade or other bodybuilders can follow various existing programs because it is their whole lives. If your daily activities are only dedicated for exercising, then you cannot find a job to meet daily needs, except those who are successful in bodybuilding for living.

Do not forget that many of them use steroids to be like that.

While you or me or most people have other activities beyond that, thus we may not be able to follow the exercise and dietary patterns every day.

That is why we stop....
THAT IS WHY WE GIVE UP.

But what if I say that there is an alternative way that may change all that.

LET ME INTRODUCE YOU TO MD

Although some will say that MD will become a trend that will disappear like most diets do. Others will say that we have to watch and see if this diet plan will survive into the future or just be a temporary fad.

But honestly; ask yourself this question.
 Has anyone of you ever managed to withstand any diet you have tried for any length of time? At most, maybe only 10% from all of us have had the kind of success we wanted.
It's basically a choice.

Can you endure eating brown rice with chicken breast or egg white everyday for any significant amount of time? Only you can answer that. For me it's the best and easiest way.
So again, it's a matter of a choice my friend.

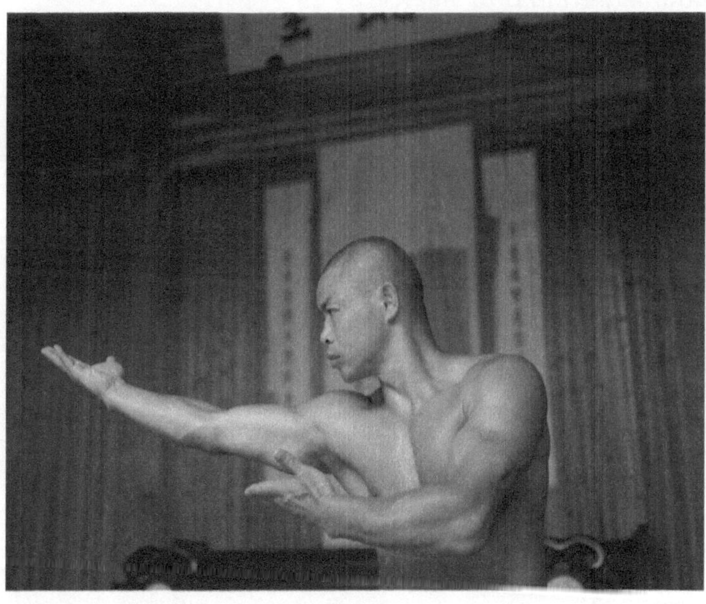

INFORMATION:

- In the first week of publication, 2 million copies of this eBook had been downloaded.

- Within that first week, many suppliers of supplement products contacted me to discuss the "contradictions"contained in the book.

- Within a week, thousands, EVEN A MILLION people were experiencing changes in their body shape.

THIS HAS BECOME A PHENOMENON! IT IS LOVED AND TALKED ABOUT BY SO MANY BECAUSE IT SIMPLY WORKS!

According to a survey done by record holder republic, MD has performed for more than 4 million people within a period of 3 weeks.

Even many artists have been successful and happy with MD because finally they can eat delicious food again and maintain their body shape!!
 That's how good MD is.

THIS IS Monks Diet

In a nutshell, MD is fasting.

. . . While continuing to eat and drink.

WHAT?!? (You say)

Don't shy away when you hear the word "fasting."This fasting enables you to eat any time and eat whatever you want.

BUT BEFORE EXPLAIN HOW LET WE READ THIS FIRST.

"Everyone has a physician inside him or her; we just have to help it in its work. The natural healing force within each one of us is the greatest force in getting well. Our food should be our medicine. Our medicine should be our food. But to eat when you are sick is to feed your sickness." – Hippocrates

and:

"Instead of using medicine, rather fast a day." – Plutarch

Do you know why almost all religion teaches their followers to fast?

Yeah, besides the religious need?

That was the first question to me by the taxi driver.

Apart from that question, this is what I found on my search.

The roots of this type of diet may have existed before

human life originated.

In Buddhism,this is known as the Theravada tradition.

This is the tradition of Theravada monks:

Abstain from taking food at a specific time.

This means that when following the tradition of Theravada monks, the rules are that on a specific day, the monks do not eat from noon to sunrise in the next day.

Fasting in the monastic community is regarded as an ascetic practice, a "dhutanga".

Dhutanga, translated means "patience and meditation training."
Dhutanga is a specific list of rules for engaging in meditation.

One of them reads:

One-sessioner's practice (ekasanik'anga) – eating one meal a day and refusing other food offered before midday. (Those Gone Forth may not, unless ill, partake of food from midday until dawn the next day). Eat once a day at noon.

Let's take it another step forward.
 In Islam, FASTING is done in the Holy Ramadan month, and one form of fasting known as:

PROPHET DAVID FASTING

David fasting is the most popular fasting to date.

This fasting is special because if you study history you will know that the Prophet David was not only a prophet, but also a soldier, king and a leading war expert.
The Prophet David is a famous prophet who beat an enemy of the Philistines named Goliath.

According to his understanding, David's fasting can be interpreted as sunnah fasting which is done by fasting for a day, then breaking it in a day.
This fasting is the most Afdhal sunnah fasting and there is no other afdhal fasting besides that.

This fasting is done continuously on an ongoing basis and only bounded by one day pause. So, one day one fasts and the next day not, and so on.

In a hadith, the Prophet Muhammad said, **"Then you fast for a day and break the fast a day, this is (called) David fasting. And this is the most afdhal fasting. Then I (Abdullah bin Amrura) said: "Truly I was able to fast more that that", then the Prophet SAW said: "There is no fasting more afdhal than that." (HR Bukhari)**

And in America this is known as Eat Stop Eat.

SO IMAGINE THAT THERE IS NOTHING NEW IN THIS CASE. EVERYTHING HAS BEEN TAUGHT SINCE OUR ANCESTORS.

What you will learn from my book is not new, but has been proven for a long time.

SCIENTIFIC FACT ABOUT

Approximately 3-4 hours after we eat, we enter what is known as postabsorbtive condition, where insulin starts to drop.

This is where the energy used by the body starts to come into internal sources in body.

The liver is the major source of stored glycogen through glycogenolysis (remember, the main source is not from muscle, but fat unless they are involved in hard activity or once your fat levels fall below 7%).

Also with insulin falling (and a drop in blood sugar) comes an increase in lipolysis (the release of fat for use as energy) and gluconeogensis (converting the sources of non-carbohydrates such as glycerol and amino acidsto glucose).

The level of lipolytic hormones such as glucagon, HGH (growth hormone) and catecholamines would increase (alsothe body's sensitivity to them) **which allows more fat to be released when doing MD.**

The longer people go without food (low state of insulin / lowered blood sugar), the more this process is increased.

A perfect example is when we go to bed and sleep without eating at night.
Most of the time our heart works to supply blood to our brain (glucose hog) with the process of burning glycogen and fat.

This situation will continue to occur up to 3 days without eating and then if it is continued, it will, bit by bit, damage the body.

But when it is limited to a maximum time of 48 hours then the benefits you'll get can be incredible.

In short, **fasting for a short time (a state without food) can cause the body to burn fat much faster.**

This short term fasting increases lipolysis. (the process of releasing fat.)
 This is done by lowering insulin and increasing lipolytic hormones (such as glucagon, growth hormone and catecholamines).

Fat cells get a strong message to open their doors for burning.

Not everyone agrees with this ..why?

NUTRITION EXPERT PROTEST

Unfortunately, many people will start complaining at this time without reading further .. Usually they (especially bodybuilders and nutritionists) will begin to make statements such as the following:

1. If you are fasting then you will deplete muscle tissue (muscle will be lost)

2. If you are fasting then you will damage and decrease your metabolism

3. If you are fasting then you will be lacking in protein intake and so on.

4. We have to eat small portions 6 times a day to maintain metabolism and build muscle

5. Protein intake should be plentiful and done immediately or your muscle will not develop.

My question is...

Where did you get a theory like this? Reading?
Googling? Or gossip?

Did you know that the contemporary caricature of
Santa Clause was first created by the 18th and 19th
century writers Washington Irving, Clement Clarke
Moore, historian John Pintard and illustrator Thomas
Nast? Probably not!

Same with this.
How can you know? Most of it comes from casual
conversation.   Many   will   assert   that:

THERE IS NO RESEARCH TO CONFIRM THAT THIS IS
TRUE. IF SO, WHEN WAS THE RESEARCH DONE AND
BY WHO?

BUT DID YOU KNOW THAT RESEARCHIS NOT THE
ABSOLUTE AND THAT IT IS GROWING EVERY DAY? A
THEORY A CAN BE POSTULATED IN A SHORT AMOUNT
OF TIME. IT'S THE SAME WITH MY OWN THEORY.

LET'S TAKE A LOOK AT THIS THEORY: (part 1)

Not eating at all is different from fasting

**Research in fact has demonstrated that with up
to 72 hours of fasting, the metabolism will not
slow down. (Macdonald IA, Webber J, 1995), and
instead it slightly improves the metabolism. Yes!
That's what I said! It will increase! (It is after
the 72-hour period that will cause it to
decrease).**

This means that short-term fasting by its self will not
lower your metabolism.

As long as you do not fast without eating at all for a long period of time you will be fine and it will increase your metabolism.

It is true that in the long run, there is a higher risk for loss of muscle mass, but if fasting is done correctly and not for an extended period of time you will not lose muscle tissue.

Your body's tendency in fact is to maintain and retain muscle. There are several different hormonal signals that cause you retain muscle and increase your metabolism.

Growth hormone (GH) is one of the hormones involved in lipolysis that increases with fasting.

HGH has a **"muscle saving"** property as well and most of the studies demonstrated that through fasting, people do not lose muscle mass in an environment of elevated HGH.

In one study (Norrelund H et al, 2001) a test group underwent 40 hoursin a state of starving by eating a low calorie diet /nutrition demonstrated that their bodies began to deteriorate and decline in health.

You can starve by eating 6 times a day if your calorie intake is too low.

(Try eating only one or two crackers every 2 hours 6 times a day. Hungry, are you not?)It has nothing to do with the frequency of your meals, justthe total calories you take in for longer periods of time (in terms of days, or weeks).

So if you miss a few hours between meals, it's still scary when you think you will be sick if you don't eat, or think that because you are unhealthy orjust because of mental pressure you cannot resist eating?

Your metabolism will drop and then you'll get even fatter! This is another fear.

And let's not forget the myth that says eating more frequently will speed up your metabolism.

It's about the total calorie intake, and how long you go without food, not meal frequency.
EATING IS EATING. THE IMPORTANT THING IS THE NUMBER OF CALORIES YOU CONSUME, NOT WHEN YOU EAT OR WHAT YOU EAT! (I don't get into the debate about eating healthy or not. It's the amount of calories that's important.)

Simply,calories are calories, regardless of their form they are still just calories. If you eat 30 pieces of apple the calories are higher than the calories in fried rice with egg.

LET'S TAKE A LOOK AT THIS THEORY: (part 2)

"But they say that when you fast you will lose MUSCLE!"

Do you really think your body's internal survival mechanism is so stupid that it will take only your muscle tissue directly and not defend it?

Let me ask you...

If your right hand is broken and in a cast and your left hand is normal, and you eat the same food every day for a month and after a month, what happens?

You cut the plaster off of your hand and what do you discover? What happens?

Which hand will lose muscle mass? Right hand or left?

Yes! Your right hand with CAST will shrink, right? That means whatever youeat it will remain smaller because there is no external stimulus such as motion or exercise! Our body is smart.

"Some nutritionists claim that the levels of your testosterone maybe decreased during fasting."

Testosterone is very important for the growth of muscle in the human body both for men and for women.

In women the level is smaller so women should not be afraid of gaining large amounts of muscle like men do when they are lifting weights.
But is it true that when fasting these levels will decrease?

Many athletes resort to using testosterone injections to build muscle mass and reduce fat. Consequently it is believed that fasting can reduce testosterone levels. In fact, testosterone will increase 20% - 30% in the morning when people wake up.

This means that the levels increase not when we eat but while we sleep.

The level of testosterone has long been observed to have little if no connection with dieting. When a person reduces caloric intake by 15% it has been shown not to interfere with testosterone at all in healthy humans.

Other studies say that rising levels of fat are associated with decreased testosterone levels or that higher levels of fat can possibly reduce testosterone levels.

This is frequently interpreted to mean that if we reduce fat, we can raise our testosterone levels.

In a study of obese people who are dieting using reduced caloric intake it was shown that they exhibited lower testosterone levels than people who eat normally.

This research was not accompanied with exercise.

So what happens is simply the process of starvation.

Starvation process is different from the concept of fasting.

Remember, that fasting is never intended to starve a person because starvation is a system designed to reduce the intake of calories.

It is true that testosterone levels will decrease slightly when a person fasts for 58 to 84 hours, but is only slightly reduced and is considered still within normal levels.

It will not make significant change if you do not fast more than 9 full days without incoming caloric intake.

It has been proven that fasting for a short time does not have a negative effect on testosterone levels.

"Eating 6 times a day with a few calories is better than 1 or 2 times with a large intake of calories."

You've no doubt heard it from multiple sources that if you eat 6 times a day it is better for burning calories, provides adequate protein and also preserves muscle mass.

Most of this theory says that if we eat 6 times a day with smaller quantities of calories, the metabolism and energy expenditure will be improved.

Actually, if we want to investigate further, this idea possibly originated from the hypothesis of a man named J. V. Neel.

In his research called The Thrifty Genotype, this study has been interpreted and developed by many researchers and is also often misunderstood.
This hypothesis states that humans have a survival mechanism that stores fat to be used in an emergency.

 From this study, many concluded that with small but frequent intake of calories, 6 times, then energy consumption will be improved, because when people do not feel hungry then the fat will not be stored and will be burned instead. (Survival Systems do not feel the need foremergency backupfat because the intake is always good) According to me this is wrong! Survival is survival.

Whatever number of meals you eat,whenever you eat, and as often as you eat, your bodywill still store fat for an emergency

People with a weekly pay day will still have the same savings as people who receive their pay on a monthly basis if they make the effort to save their money.

Our bodies will keep storing fat for emergencies and do not care about the amount, the time or the frequency.
The fat reserves will be used when the humans really need it.
Have you ever heard stories of people stranded at sea without food, and yet they lived?

That and other events when food becomes scarce is when food reserves in the form of fat are used.
It is in these types of events when human survival depends on the amount of fat in there is in reserve.

I ask you, what with the current state of your life in a city where food is everywhere and food intake is 6 times a day, where is the state of stress that causes your body to use up its reserves of fat?

 It isn't there! In the mean time your body continues to save up fat for an emergency.

 Fasting on the other hand simulates the state of stress.
From this we can draw the conclusion that eating 6 times a day will only make your bodystore fat continually whileanticipating the emergency where it will be needed.

THE RIGHT KIND OF FASTING

THE RIGHT KIND OF FASTING WILL INCREASE YOUR HGH WHICH WILL MAKE YOU YOUNGER AND MORE MUSCULAR!!

Go without food for several hours will NOT slow down your metabolism!

It will not cause havoc your blood sugar. Short term fasting will improve insulin sensitivity and this is a huge advantage.

When your cells are sensitive to insulin, they do a better job working with your pancreas. Loss of insulin sensitivity creates a risk factor for heart disease, diabetes and obesity as well!

Short Fasting also reduces oxidative stress and inflammation of the cells. It helps in the repair of DNA damage that can develop into cancer. In fact research shows that fasting slows down our aging clock. Fasting can help us live longer and help to keep our organs youthful.

This is from Wikipedia:

Extended fasting has been recommended as therapy for various conditions by health professionals of most cultures, throughout history, from ancient to modern.

Research suggests there are major health benefits to caloric restriction. Benefits include reduced risks of cancer, cardiovascular diseases, diabetes, insulin resistance, immune disorders and more generally, the slowing of the aging process, and the potential to increase maximum life span. Besides these health benefits, research by Valter Longo has also uncovered a potential link between fasting and improved efficacy of chemotherapy.

WOW!!

As you can see this is true from ancient times. But we never realize why, what or how to manipulate this fasting method to give us more of the results we need for our body.

Did you know that Plato and Aristotle said that to stop eating for short periods of time, i.e. fasting is a drug for any disease including cancer?

Human Trial(s)

In 2009 there was a case study that delivered some promising results. Ten cancer patients – four with breast cancer, two with prostate cancer, one each with ovarian, lung, uterine, and esophageal cancers – underwent fasting prior to and after chemotherapy treatment. Fasting times ranged from 48-140 hours prior to and 5-56 hours after; all were effective at reducing side effects of chemotherapy.

In the first case, a 51-year old woman with breast cancer did her first round of chemotherapy in a fasting state for 140 hours. Other than dry mouth, fatigue, and hiccups, she felt well enough to go to work andresume her normal daily activities. For the subsequent two rounds, she did not fast and instead ate hernormal diet, and the side effects were extremely pronounced – severe fatigue, diarrhea, weakness,abdominal pain, nausea – and they prevented her from returning to work.

For her fourthround of chemotherapy,she fasted, and the side effects were again minimized. And it wasn't just the subjective effects that improved with fasting, but also her physiological markers. Total white blood cell, absolute neutrophil counts, and platelet counts were all highest after the fasting regimens.

The point is fasting is a good thing when done properly and right. Is it no wonder that almost all religions teach it?

The question is how does this MD fast work, where you can still eat delicious food,eat at any hour you want and eat what you wantbut you are still fasting and can have your dream body?

This is the real secret of the monk's fasting; or better yet, any Fasting!

Sometimes an ancient message can be easily forgotten.

Then again how can you fast, where you can eat delicious food, eat what you want, at any time, anywhere?

Monks Diet Fasting Methods

Now the part you've all been waiting for

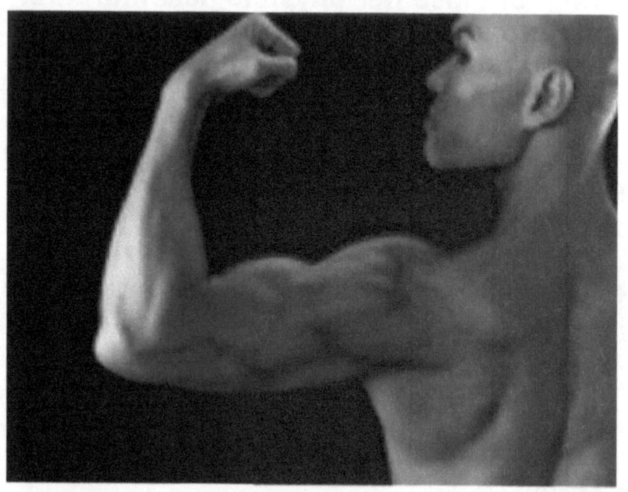

A great body isn't made just in the exercise gym with supplements alone.

Ask any health expert, they all will say same thing. Creating a great body isn't done only in the gym.

Only 30% of the job of creating a great physique is accomplished through exercise, although without that 30% you cannot build the great body you want, the other 70% is accomplished through your mouth.

You are what you eat.

What you are also **depends on how much you eat and When you eat!**

Therefore, there are two certain factors in the formation of our bodies:

1. If you take in more calories than you use up, your body will store the extra calories in the form of fat.

2. If you take in fewer calories than you use up, your body will burn up the fat.
How do I pull out calorie?

Well, whatever you doing, even if you are sleeping, you are burning calories. This is called resting metabolism.

Now let's explore how the implementation of MD into your daily life forms the shape of your body!

THE MONK'S SECRET OF FASTING

I will start with

MD BREAKFAST (Break fasting)

Dinner is okay, but breakfast? NO! NO! NO!

Let's toss out a really pernicious myth before we do anything else. Let's talk about breakfast.

How many of you have heard that breakfast is the most important meal in a day?

Have you heard that the advantage of breakfast is that it will give you energy and make you not want to eat more during lunch and there by help to maintain your body?

If you search the internet you can find 1001 reasons why you should eat breakfast, and still not come to the end of it.

If you get this down, and listen to my words,

everything will change.

Have you noticed that some little children don't like to eat breakfast in the morning?

 Do you remember as a child, being upset because you were forced to eat breakfast?

As time went on, you grew accustomed to it.
Why is it that little children frequently don't like to eat breakfast?

Do you remember being upset when you were little and told to eat your breakfast?

Did you know that among children who eat a big breakfast in the morning, 90% of them are overweight?

 Do you remember being sleepy in class and even hungry at your first break at school after you've eaten breakfast???

Believe it or not, eating breakfast will make you hungry all day long. It will make you sleepy all day long. What is more, it will lower your fat burning capacity when compared to skipping dinner.

"But I stopped eating dinner and I keep losing weight!," you scream.

Yes, yes. I know.

You lose weight not because of the dinner itself, but because you have reduced 1 part of your daily meals. It's just that simple.

If you didn'teat dinner the intake of calories is not

increased. Consequently, the myth that says eating dinner makes you fat is wrong!

Dinner simply means that you are adding one more meal, hence the added calories. Calories cannot tell time. If your calorie intake is 2000, skipping dinner, lunch, or breakfast is exactly the same.

If you burn only 1500 calories during that same day it means you have an extra 500 calories for your body to store as fat. When you stopped eating dinner, you lost weight. OF COURSE! It's because you reduced the amount of calorie intake. **Get it?**

Remember when you ate a lot and you became sleepy?

On the other hand, if you have dinner it's good to sleep, because when you sleep, you are still burning calories.

SO WHY STOP EATING BREAKFAST INSTEAD OF DINNER?

"So how about breakfast?" you ask.

Almost everybody teaches that you should not eat a late breakfast. They will tell you that breakfast is beneficial, that it gives you energy, that you need it for your activity, that it builds your metabolism, makes your muscles healthy, feeds your brain and helps you concentrate all day long and . . . BLAH-BLAH-BLAAAAAH . . . YADA-YADA-YADA.

What if this is all wrong?

And this is new research information about breakfast.

Breakfast is a meal consumed after we get out of bed and before we become active.

If you eat at 2PM and you got out of bed at 1PM, and not at 8AM, that's a breakfast, right?

What is the meaning of the word "breakfast"? **Break fast; not just eating in the morning.**

The following is the research result:

Studies [citation and reference needed here, otherwise just say "Common sense demonstrates" instead of "Studies show"] show that people eat the same size meals at lunch and dinner regardless of how much they eat at breakfast. This means that whether or not people eat breakfast, the quantity of lunch and dinner will be the same. It doesn't mean that if you eat breakfast you will reduce the amount of food at lunch and dinner like the nutrition experts say.

This challenges the controversial wisdom that says that if you skip breakfast, you will be very hungry and eat more food at lunch.

The quantity of your meals is not based on whether or not you have already eaten or not but instead it has to do with your personal habits. If you are already accustomed to eating like a pig, you will continue the same habit, regardless of whether or not you've had breakfast.

Have you ever seen a skinny person who didn't have time to eat one meal, and then at the next meal eats like there's no tomorrow? Seriously, I doubt you have. Have you have seen fat people eat this way? WELL!

Previously there was research done in October of 2012; a study performed at Imperial College London, comparing the brain scans and calorie intake of 21 people who ate or skipped breakfast. Medical News Today summarized the findings: "Skipping breakfast increases hunger, the attraction of high food calorie and food intake at lunch."

What happened?
Psychological bias, that's what.
Imagine you were in a research program that didn't allow you to eat breakfast.

At lunch they serve you a sumptuous meal, rich in calories. What will you do unconsciously without even thinking about it?

Who can resist a free meal? You will eat as much as possible. After all, you are eating on someone else's dime, and your brain is telling you to indulge as an act of revenge.

It isn't your stomach doing the talking!
 Remember, they are thinking that this is legitimate research, but without realizing it they expect it to demonstrate that you will overeat when you've had no breakfast.

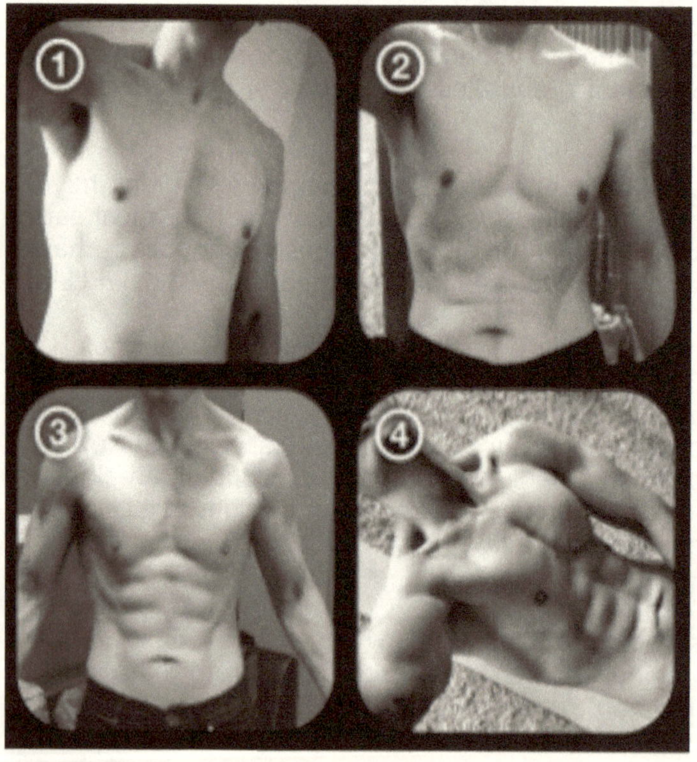

Some claim that skipping breakfast will cause obesity. Ha-ha-ha! Obesity is not caused by breakfast, lunch or dinner! Watch how an obese person eats. It's a matter of habit!

Another study recently explored the difference between engaging in exercise withfull or an empty stomach.

At the end of January, the British Journal of Nutrition published a paper that suggests that exercise before breakfastburns 20 percent more body fat than the same exercise after breakfast.
The study also determined that people who exercise before breakfast did not consume extra calories or experience increased appetiteduring the day.

These are the NEW Facts!

Doctor Javier Gonzalez, a member of the research team, told Science Daily: "In order to lose body fat we need access our stored fat and use it for energy. If exercise is done after an overnight fast without breakfast we will increase the total amount of energy burned, and make the larger proportion come from the burning of our excess of stored energy in the form of fat."

You may have heard a study that said people who eat breakfast, have a healthier, thinner body compared with those who did not eat breakfast.
You may have also heard that avoiding breakfast will make you fat. This makes me laugh when I hear it especially when it comes from a well known nutritionist. Never in my life have I ever seen a fat person avoid breakfast, lunch or dinner.

It is true there is research to support that people who eat breakfast are healthier than those who do not. But these studies take samples of people who eat breakfast over the long term versus people who do not. This means that there is a serious bias in studies of this kind.

What do I mean by bias?

Bias means that important factors are being ignored. People who are the subjects of the study are the ones whose regular lifestyle already includes breakfast and not breakfast skipping lifestyle.
The bias is that the subjects who eat a regular breakfast tend to be those from a well educated, economically prosperous class who care more about their weight as opposed to those who are from a lower income class who work a lot of overtime and don't have the time to think about or care about their weight.
Right from the start, a different economical lifestyle places a random but important factor that is not accounted for in the study. The study is done on a voluntary basis and people with the same lifestyle participating in this kind of study are not taken into account.

Think about how many packaged breakfast product producers benefit from "research" that supports the sales of their products.

So to answer the premise that avoiding breakfast will make you overeat at lunch for me is funny because we are making a conscious decision and not by accident or by forgetting it. Secondly, even if it's true that we eat more lunch and dinner, commonly the total calorie intake is still reduced. I personally have concluded that skipping breakfast is not harmful.

In conclusion, breakfast will rob you of the opportunity to burn off extra fat energy by starting your morning exercise after your overnight fast. Whereas dinner energy will burn off while you sleep and doesn't create a problem.

7 Reasons Skipping breakfast

Here are 7 reasons why you do not need breakfast

1.Breakfast doesn't increase your metabolism

Studies have demonstrated that fasting or not eating breakfast has no effect on metabolism. Eating consistently every 3 hours and including breakfast also has no measurable effect.

2.Breakfast will not help you maintain muscle mass.

Maintaining muscle mass has more to do with exercise than with your meals. You will not lose muscle if you don't eat every 3 hours. You sleep for 6 to 8 hours every night and doesn't cause muscle loss does it? Your muscles don't need protein every 3 hours while they are resting.

3. Breakfast is managing your blood sugar.

The general idea is that breakfast increases your blood sugar and assists in helping to control your insulin levels. Insulin is the key to muscle growth but it is also involved with fat storage.

Fasting is more useful for reducing insulin levels and dramatically improving the cellular sensitivity for insulin. This is far more important.

4.Breakfast increases hunger.

Many people, including myself feel hungry during the day after eating breakfast.

It could be a benefit or a drawback, depending on whether you wantgain muscle weight or lose fat.

To add weight:
If you're a skinny guy who fights foreating a lot, eating breakfast will make it easier to achieveyour calorie needs.

For fat loss: more frequent meals are of no benefit. The hunger we feel during the day is a state of mind that you experience whether or not you eat breakfast. Remember that if you don't eat in the morning, you have fat that can be burned instead.

For me and a lot of people eating breakfast creates an addiction to food and makes you want to eat again. This means calories added that can easily cause you to have a surplus of calories that will be converted into fat.

5. Breakfast does not make you healthier

People who do not eat breakfast are typically the ones who don't exercise and eat donuts on their way to work, eat junk food during the day and eat a big dinner in front of the TV.

These are people who don't want to diet.
They're not eating breakfast, but they are trading it instead with a snacking habit, and this is clearly unhealthy.

Those of us who are working to lose weight and improve our health don't do this because we know which habits are good and which ones are not.

Breakfast is not beneficial to your health directly, but it does help to establish healthy eating habits. Studies claim that breakfast and health condition does not have a direct correlation.

Breakfast does not properly manage blood sugar.
Breakfast does not increase your metabolism.
Breakfast does not prevent muscle damage.
Breakfast can make you hungry in the rest of the day.

6.Breakfast can even disrupt concentration

Studies suggest fasting for 48 hours did not affect cognitive tests negatively.
You do not need breakfast for your mental alertness.

Many people, especially students will skip breakfast because they know they will be more productive, concentrate better and be more motivated for the rest of the day.
 This is also my personal experience.

7. Breakfast certainly not natural

Our ancestors probably did not eat a big breakfast: Before they could eat they had to hunt it down first. For a hunter, a small lunch and a big dinner is more the natural norm.

Did you remember when you were little and you hated to eat breakfast?
BUT YOUR PARENTS FORCED YOU? This is because breakfast is created **BY SOCIAL FACTORS NOT HUMAN INSTINCT!**

7 Reasons Skipping breakfast : Proof

Here are Proof why you do not need breakfast

Skipping breakfast is much better than skipping dinner.
This is something I want to make perfectly clear.

Remember that almost all of the articles that say that skipping breakfast can cause disease etc. frequently add a disclaimer in the fine print that states that the correlation of this study is not clear.
You can check this for yourself :
The following link contains samples of articles that say skipping breakfast can have negative consequences:

http://www.usatoday.com/story/news/nation/2013/07 /22/skipping-breakfastheart-attack-risk/2575723/

The contents:

ATLANTA — Another reason to eat breakfast: Skipping it may increase your chances of a heart attack.

A study of older men found those who regularly skipped breakfast had a 27% higher risk of a heart attack than those who ate a morning meal. **There's no reason why the results wouldn't apply to other people, too, the Harvard researchers said.**

Other studies have suggested a link between breakfast and obesity, high blood pressure, diabetes and other health problems seen as precursors to heart problems.

"But no studies looked at long-term risk of heart attack," said Eric Rimm, one of the study authors at the Harvard School of Public Health.

Why would skipping breakfast be a heart attack risk?

Experts aren't certain, but here's what they think: People who don't eat breakfast are more likely to be hungrier later in the day and eat larger meals. Those meals mean the body must process a larger amount of calories in a shorter amount of time. That can spike sugar levels in the blood and perhaps lead to clogged arteries.

But is a stack of syrupy pancakes, greasy eggs and lots of bacon really better than eating nothing?

Why I Skip Breakfast to Maintain my Weight

Follow > Alzheimer's, The Balanced Life, Aging Gracefully, Aging Gracefully, Weight Loss, Healthy Living Health News, Parkinson's Disease, Weight Loss Tips, Alzheimer's Disease, Anti-Aging, Cardiovascular Disease, Fasting, How To Lose Weight, Intermittent Fasting, Longevity, Losing Weight, Weight, Work-Life Balance, Canada Living News

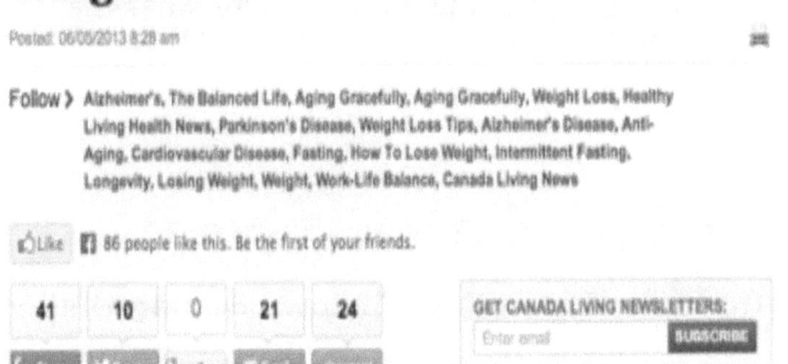

researchers did not ask what the study participants ate for breakfast, and were not prepared to pass judgment on whether a fatty, sugary breakfast is better than no breakfast at all.

Other experts agreed that it's hard to say.

*"We don't know whether it's the timing or content of breakfast that's important. It's probably both,"*said Andrew Odegaard, a University of Minnesota researcher who has studied a link between skipping breakfast and health problems like obesity and high blood pressure."

"Generally, people who eat breakfast tend to eat a healthier diet," he added.

The new research was released Monday by the journal Circulation. It was an observational study, so it's not designed to prove a cause and effect.

Try to read the underlined statements above, they even doresearch but they are not sure what they are doing and their what the correlation is. Now that's FUNNY.

Eating Window : Fasting Limit

Introducing The Eating Window : Fasting Limit

After stop eat breakfast, I will introduce you to eating window.

Fasting with limited eating time and eat anything without thinking about calories.

Keep in mind that this does not mean you can suddenly become greedy and eat blindly.
 Many think that after fast they can eat as much as they want.

 This wrong!

 Eat normally like you eat each day.
Don't think about what you eat. Just eat your usual meal.

MD WILL NOT SUCCEED IF YOU BECOME GREEDY AFTER FASTING UNLESS YOU ARE IN THE ENLARGEMENT PHASE OF YOUR BODY. (I will discussed this problem later) THIS ALSO MEANS THAT YOU MUST NOT BECOME GREEDY.

Fasting here means there must not be any calorie intake.

You can drink water, tea or eat **anything so long as it has no calories**. You can even eat candy with 0 calories.
NO FRUIT or MILK OR VEGETABLES.

Someone asked me once if they could drink milk or eat fruit or vegetables during a fast.
 My answer . . . Can you sleep with you eyes open?
You can, but you are not really sleeping if you do.
Fasting is like that. If you eat something with calories in it, your fast has falled.

Why is this so important? Because MD is a diet with emphasis on HGH (discussed later) that emerges when there is no calorie intake for 16 hours. So if you take in any calories, even in a small amount, you FAIL!

FASTING TIME

The fasting time I gave is 16 hours, 18 hours and 20 hours (time without food).

This means the meal time is 8 hours, 6 hours and 4 hours also called the eating window.

What does that mean?

This means you may eat whatever you usually eat (**don't be suddenly greedy**) for 4, 6 or 8 hours a day (without having breakfast at least 3 or 4 hours after you wake up)

So if you abide by an 8 hour window it means that you start eating at 12PM until 8PM, 3 meals, or if you start eating at 3PM, you can eat to 12 AM.

If you utilize a 6 hour window, you eat at 12 PM with your last meal at 6PM. There is no restriction on when you start your eating time. It's all up to you.

If you take 4 hours eating time and start eat at 2PM, you can eat till 6 PM.

You can eat many times when you feel hungry but not eat blindly! The magic is you will not feel hungry.

This is the first kind of fasting.

With this fast you can set your own eating timewhen you have dinner party or at a later time.

Very flexible!

REMEMBER MD WILL FAIL IF YOU EAT BLINDLY AFTER YOU BREAK MD FASTING.

Eating Window : Fasting 24 hours

Introducing The Eating Window : Fasting 24 hours

This is the second type.
It sounds scary, right?

This means you only eat once a day.
You can eat any time, whatever you want and however many as you want.

Don't eat blindly don't eat breakfast, and while fasting you can drink non calorie liquids.
Assume you start eating on Wednesday (tentative day) at 3 PM, eat one substantial meal.

That's it! You can drink whatever you want as long as it has no calories.

Only eat once on Wednesday till the next day on Thursday at 3 PM then you are into your eating window.

For example you choose a 4 hour window so you can eat on Thursday from 3 PM till 7 PM.
That's fasting 24 hours.

Do you remember that one time in your life when you ate only one meal?
The question that usually arises is: "Will that cause dizziness, headaches or other problems?

NOT when you grow accustomed to it. Maybe in the very beginning when you are unfamiliar, but after 2 tries then the problems will disappear.
Remember to take in enough calories when in your window so that you will not be dizzy.

Example:
If you eat 6 times, but you only eat crackers, you will be stressed out and dizzy.
If you eat once a day but 2 portions of lemak rice with enough calories for one day and you will get through the day without any problems.

CAUTION:

Basically, women only need about 1200-1500 calories a day and men 2000-2500 a day, so if you eat more than that it will fatten you regardless of the kind of food, and eating less than that will make you slimmer.
For example fried rice has 750 calories. If you eat 2 portions it's already enough to fill your day.

So if you have enough calories you will not feel sick or dizzy when you eat only once a day.
What if you have ulcer?
Talk to your doctor about it, but you can break your fast with your liquid ulcer treatment.

Remember that most of the time ulcers are caused by your own thoughts. If in your mind you are in agreement, it will be okay

Combined implementation between your eating window and fasting 24 hours.

Simple....

Your Eating window

In the first week you have to start with your window of eating 8 hours a day without breakfast. This will be easy for you.

In the second week, narrow your window down to 6 hours a day.

In third week and beyond your eating window will be 4 hours a day.

Remember you can stop at 8 hours a day for the rest of your life or at 6 hours if you want without having to go to 4 hours a day but if you do, the results will not be maximized.

You will need a longer time for slimming or building your body if you are stuck at 8 hours or 6 hours.

When I began fasting, I entered the 4 hours a day window in the second week.

You can do this for as long as you wish even for your whole life.

If you prefer, you can stay at the 8 hour window. That means you only skip breakfast. A child can do that.

If you start with the 4 hour a day window, that's EXTRAORDINARY! Congratulations!
If you prefer, you can alternate.

For example over the period of a week you can open windows to eat 8 hours on Saturday or Sunday and the rest only 4 hours.

And there are more alternatives you can take.

As long as you stick to the rules it works, just not as quickly. But if you can stay with the 4 hour window every day, this will produce extraordinary results in a short time.

24 Hour Fasting.

If you want to get better and faster results you can put aside one or two days out of the week for a 24 hour fast. I do this three days out of the week.

Don't be afraid. This doesn't mean you don't eat at all. As I said, do you remember ever in your life saying, "wow, I just ate once today,"? You must have... and you can.

Suppose you ateat 4 PM then ate again the next day starting at 4 PM again and entered your eating window patterns as in the first example above.

Very easy.

Combine those two things and your body will shape up in a short time!

Your body will become a natural fat burning machine!

MY WAY

How did I do that?

This is the sample program I did personally at the start of my program and made it a habit.

- In the first week I implemented a 6 hour eating window (an 8 hour window was too easy for me)

- In the second week I entered a 4 hour eating window. I failed on this occasionally, but the next day I went right back to the 4 hour window.

- In the third week I entered 24 hour fasting pattern once a week and combined that with a 4 hour window.

- From the fourth week until the present, I have been using a 24 hour fasting pattern twice a week with a 6 or 4 hour window.

Remember this is so very flexible!

Sometimes I only fasting once 24 hours fasting in a week with 6 hours eating window, sometimes twice with 4 hours eating window or 8 hours eating window etc.

IS THIS GREAT, OR WHAT?

Obviously without my having to explain it, you already know that the best pattern is a 4-hour window with with a 24 hour fast 2 or three times a week.
This means I can use this combination for a maximum effect. Keep in mind, nobody's perfect, but that's okay.

Within 45 to 60 days of doing this I could feel a remarkable difference in my body.
You can see it in my photographs.

I started all of this with an existing ulcer. As far as I can tell, it's gone. I was breaking my fasts starting with the ulcer medication in the first week. Now, it's gone even when I do a 24 hour fast. I discussed this earlier.

EAT, PRAY AND LOVE

Let's talk about what creates well developed muscles.
Is it supplements?
Is it exercise?
If not, what?
Let's look first at supplements.

For starters, the only supplements that have been proven in research to be effective are those containingcreatine.
Yes that's all and I will discuss that in detail later on.
Whereas your body needs protein it's not as much as you might think.

There is literature out in the culture stating that the intake of protein will keep your body muscular.
 This is incorrect if it doesn't include muscle exercise.

The truth is that the food we eat on a regular basis contains enough protein for our bodies. It's okay if you want to increase your protein intake with a supplement, but don't overdo it.

Don't waste your time thinking about protein or supplements unless you are into full bodybuilding and you are into the use of steroids.

Keep in mind that protein shakes and other supplements that contain protein also contain calories that can be stored as fat and increase your weight.

How often do you see people at the gym whom you know have purchased ten different types of supplements but their body shape is much like a big box with legs?

The serious bodybuilder can use the supplements with success because they count their calories. They follow an intense tasteless diet of plain brown rice and boiled chicken breast along with their supplements.

If that's the lifestyle for you, you're welcome to it. **You can stop reading and follow that lifestyle. Is that the lifestyle for me? NO, NO, and NO! I want to be free from that!**

My Ways : Muscle or Sales

SUPPLEMENTS FOR BUILDING MUSCLE OR FOR BOOSTING SALES?

Let's talk about protein shakes offered on the main menu at the gym.

If you ever been a member at gym or visited, they might have used scare tactics like this:

1. After intense weight lifting you must immediately take protein!!

2. If your body weight is 70 kilograms, you must immediately take in 140 grams of protein.

3. If you delay taking your protein your muscles will not properly recover and you will destroy muscle tissue instead of building it!

Some even say that using my methods will make your muscles disappear! Oh, really? My muscles are still here.

Emergency! Emergency! Your muscles will be lost if you don't use our protein supplement right away!

Take a look at who you hear this from. Usually it's from the trainer who is selling the supplements. Often it's from a bodybuilder with a very big and muscular body. Will they tell you whether or not they are using steroids? It's more than likely that they'll lie about it if you ask.

Protein shake supplements can help the development of muscle . . . especially if you don't eat regular food which already contains protein.

So if you don't eat any food and only drink the protein shake, that's good, but how much of it is needed?

Should you drink it immediately after exercise, or should you drink it every 3 hours?

The answer is NOT!

Let me explain:

More protein doesn't mean more muscle.

Protein is important for muscle development but it doesn't mean that only eat more or drink protein supplements will make muscle bigger.

So the question is; How much protein does your body need?

Look at the research. You can google it. The recommended protein intake 0.8 grams per kilogram of adult body weight.

Simply expressed, to avoid muscle loss, women need at least 46 grams of protein a day and men need at least 56 grams of protein a day.

This is far lower than what you hear out there from other people or from most nutritionists.
Certainly, if you exercise a lot, the suggested daily dose of protein will need to be increased.

What is also important to remember that the overall calorie intake also increased with the level of activity. So basically, the more you do your activity so the more total calories needed, that's the logic right?

Protein on MD

Protein on Monks Diet

Your body only absorbs about 30 grams of protein every time you eat.

How does this affect you with an MD fast, and afterwards when you eat?

 Will this cause you to loose muscle mass when you fast and eat only 2 or three times in a day, or not at all?

Most certainly NOT! Your body is far smarter than that. It will consume the fat and protein reserves and use it to build your muscle, not tear it down.

So what of the theory that says you must eat 5 or 6 times a day to keep up your protein level?

 According to the manufacturers and salespersons of Supplements it is, and if you believe them, they will love you and you will see their $mile$, as you consume their products to get your 20 grams of protein every 2-3 hours.

In reality, maybe your body works better when protein is available at random times.

The statements from Dr Eades's blog comments:

http://www.proteinpower.com/drmike/

"I don't think that protein will affect muscle mass at all. If you go without food for long periods of time, say, a few days, your metabolic system will convert your muscle mass to alter stored protein into the glucose you need to keep your blood sugar normal. BUT this doesn't happen if you fast for a short period of time."

Instead it's good to burn your fat because your muscle will use recycled junk protein from your fat!

Do you still think that you need periodic protein to build more muscle?

Here's another interesting view of how the body can actually use protein in the diet during fasting by eating only once or twice vs. eating frequently.

A research project cited in the American Journal of Clinical Nutrition, Vol. 69, No. 6, 1202-1208, June 1999 was conducted with, 15 elderly women (averaging 68 years in age), 7 of them were fed once a day for 14 days with 80% of the daily protein in the amount of 1200 calories, and the 8 remaining women were given the same amount of daily protein every 3 hours, spread over 4 meals.

The result is that there was a more positive balance of nitrogen with those who ate only once compared with those to ate more frequently.

 Muscle-forming protein turnover also higher than the group who eat more.
(American Journal of Clinical Nutrition, Vol. 69, No 6, 1202-1208, June 1999)

Consequently, the group that ate once or rarely

increased the balance of nitrogen, protein turnover and protein synthesis, compared to the ones who ate more often.

In summary they achieved a more responsive anabolic state. (muscle building state).

"Drink protein immediately after exercise and you will build muscle!" Are you sure?

(As we have heard from one source or another, if you eat immediately after exercise it will increase protein synthesis which builds muscle).

It's important to know that your body works gradually in long term and not from minute to minute. With that in mind, we should not ignore the larger overall picture of muscle recovery.

Our muscles are not built up in one hour of exercise! Our muscles can be built in 24-48 hours after exercising, while there is food intake any time.

"Even in a fed state, protein and carbohydrate supplementation stimulates muscle protein synthesis during exercise. Ingestion of protein with carbohydrate during and immediately after exercise improves whole-body protein synthesis but does not further augment muscle protein synthesis rates during 9 h of subsequent overnight recovery."

Source: Coingestion of Carbohydrate and Protein Hydrolysate Stimulates Muscle Protein Synthesis during Exercise in Young Men, with No Further Increase during Subsequent Overnight Recovery; Journal of Nutrition, doi:10.3945/jn.108.092924

This research says that there will be no additional muscle building effect in protein intake immediately after exercise.

Maybe you need direct intake if you are a bodybuilder, but I'm not. I don't think you are either, so why should you follow a bodybuilder's style which is to eat brown rice and tasteless chicken breast and bring milk anywhere you go?

THE REAL BENEFIT OF PROTEIN

Many people are using a higher protein intake because they are afraid of losing muscle. The fact is you need all different kinds of calories in order to build muscle including fat.

Why do some tell you that it is easier to lose weight with more protein?
 It's mainly because protein will make you feel full and help you to stop eating excessively.

Remember. The amount of protein you really need to build muscle is lower than what do you think, but you still need to get enough calories from your food, that's the bottom line.

I can't imagine how you enjoy life while you keep thinking about the amount of protein every time you eat . . . Hahahaha!
 Think about counting your calories while you eat. Counting calories is good thing, but it doesn't have to be a requirement at all when you eat according to what you need in MD.

MD will not make you lose any muscle, but it will utilize more internal sources (amino acids) like enzymes and unused protein in fat.

Body builders will tell you to eat 300+ grams of protein a day and exercises 5X a week.

Well, make sure you ask them what other drugs they use? Almost all body builders (not all of them) that I know have offered me steroids or pro-hormones. Well of course they need lots of protein!

The point is either you eat 1, 2 or 3 portion of food in a short time period in the eating window I told you, or 6 small portion in one full day, Your body will not have any trouble finding the best way to build muscle. In the long term, the results will be the same as long as you keep the quantity of total protein constant every day.

But it's all back to what I believe the various researches. If you want to spend a lot on protein milk, you have the right to waste your money if you want to.

How about me?

Honestly, I use **Whey protein shakes**; one glass a day as my food intake and for the purpose of building muscle.
 That's it, no more than that, which is 30 grams of protein. I do this because sometimes it's hard for me to find food in my daily life and a protein shake makes it easy to fulfill my minimum intake of daily protein.

In addition to protein, I also take 5-10 gram of Creatine before and after exercising. (**Creatine is allowed during a fast**) One of the supplements that are proven to increase strength and muscle mass in the long term is Creatine monohydrate.

And, because Creatine is not metabolized for energy and will not increase insulin levels, taking Creatine during a fast is acceptable.

Note:
In the last month I haven't used any protein shakes or Creatine and I haven't experienced any muscle decline so long as I have eaten enough food.

For convenience, women need 50 grams of protein and men need 80 grams to maintain and form their body. You can get it from the food you eat. Any more than that will not be useful.

Human Growth Hormone

So what really builds your muscles? What is it that can make your body grow rapidly? What can make you taller if you are still under 20 years old?

Yes Human Growth Hormone.

What is that?

Human growth hormone is a hormone produced by your brain which CAN restore your body's internal clock, help you to build muscle, get rid of fat, and increase your libido, while giving you tremendous energy and most amazing, it can **MAKE YOU LOOK YOUNGER AGAIN!**

Where does HGH come from?

The body naturally produces growth hormone in the pituitary gland and as the name suggests, it responsible for cell growth and regeneration.

Increasing muscle mass and bone density isn't possible without HGH, and consequently it plays a major role in maintaining the health of human tissue, including the brain and other vital organs.

When released, HGH remains active in the bloodstream for few minutes but enough for liverto turn it to growth factor. The most important is from the FORM OF INSULIN growth factor-1 or IGF-1, which offers some anabolic properties.

How can you get more HGH into the body?

There are many ways; here are a few of them:

1. HGH is released while you sleep, so you can sleep for 8-10 hours a day (not possible with my life style), but even then the HGH levels in your body will decrease soon after you reach the age of about 25 and not all people release the same amount of HGH while they sleep.

2. Incorporating artificial HGH (artificial HGH injected into your body, and there are many other supplements contain HGH. This isn't good. Why? Because your stomach can't digest HGH).

3. Fasting....

The latest research confirms the effect of fasting on human growth hormone (HGH), protein metabolism. HGH works to protect muscle and metabolic balance, a response triggered and accelerated by fasting.
During 18-24 hours fasting period, HGH increased an average 1300% in women and almost 2000% in men.

HGH INCREASED 2000% WHEN FASTING!

Let's see one more time the benefit of fasting from the point of research:

A research at Murray, UT (3/4/11), fasting decreses the risk of heart disease such astriglycerides, body weight and blood sugar level.

Fasting has long been associated with religious rituals, diets and political protests or demonstration.
Now, new evidence from cardiac researchers at Intermountain Medical Center Heart Institute shows that regular fasting is also good for your health.

Even research cardiologists at the Intermountain Medical Center Heart Institute reported that fasting not only lowered the risk of coronary arteries disease and diabetes, but also causes significant changes in cholesterol levels.

 Diabetes and high cholesterol is a risk factor for coronary heart disease.

This invention extends a research from 2007 Intermountain Healthcare research that revealed the relationship between fasting and reduction of the risk of coronary heart disease, the main cause of death among men and women in America.

In the new research, fasting was also found to reduce other cardiac risk factors, such as triglycerides, weight and blood sugar levels.

These findings were presented at the American College of Cardiology annual scientific sessions in New Orleans.

"These new conclusions suggest that our findings are not coincidence events," said Dr. Benjamin D. Home, PhD, MPH, director of cardiovascular and genetic epidemiology at Intermountain Medical Center Heart Institute, and the lead researchers in that study.

In contrast to previous research done by the team, this new research recorded the reactions in the body's biological mechanisms during the fasting period.

Participants of low-density lipoprotein cholesterol (LDL-C, "bad" cholesterol) and high-density lipoprotein cholesterol (HDL-C, "good" cholesterol), both increased (14 percent and 6 percent, respectively), increased total cholesterol and made the researchers surprised. (I WILL TALK ABOUT THIS AGAIN LATER).

"Fasting causes hunger stress. As a response, your body will release more cholesterol, allowing it to utilize fat as a source of fuel, not glucose.
This reduces the number of fat cells in the body," said Dr. Horne. "This is important because the fewer fat cells in body then the less likely you will experience insulin resistance, or diabetes." **I will discuss later that cholesterol levels do not cause heart disease**.

This new study also confirms previous findings about the effects of fasting on human growth hormone (HGH), protein metabolism.

HGH works to protect muscle and metabolic balance, a response triggered and accelerated by fasting. During an 18-24 hour fasting period, HGH increased an average of 1,300 percent in women, and nearly 2,000 percent in men.

In this latest experiment, the researchers conducted two fasting studies of over 200 people – both patients and healthy volunteers – who were recruited at Intermountain Medical Center. A second 2011 clinical trial followed by 30 patients who only drank water and did not eat anything for 24 hours.

They got blood tests and physical measurements to evaluate cardiac risk factors, markers of metabolic risk, and other general health parameters. And the results were incredible. HGH up and all body functions were getting better.

So basically by fasting you will have more HGH, which means more MUSCLE. But it only works if you are fasting in the right way.

So the point is the forming of my muscle using my boosted HGH as much as 2,000 percent..... **THAT'S THE SECRET!**

Conclusions:

1. MD is proven to be the easiest and healthiest lifestyles anybody could utilize. (For healthy individuals, not impaired by specific maladies, or pregnancy.)

2. Research shows that fasting can help prevent heart disease, cancer, diabetes and other disease and disorders.

3. Our ancestors followed this fasting lifestyle for thousands of years. This means we were created for it.

4. Recent studies show that fasting increased HGH in women up to 1,300% and in men up to 2,000%!

5. It optimizes your energy levels and your body metabolism becomes a "fat burner" so you can lose weight through normalization of insulin and leptin.

6. MD really can help you gain muscle mass without you experiencing muscle damage.

7. MD will work well if you do not become greedy and do not eat blindly after you finish fasting and is followed by exercise for maximum results.

8. Eating healthy food in MD is very good. If you have choices on your food, choose healthy food for your eating window. Reduce carbohydrates and sugar.

The Essence of MD

You can control the calories you take in by limiting your eating time, and control snacking. Without even realizing it you will limit the quantity of the calories that you take in every day.

The shorter your eating window, the more control you have over your calorie intake. Remember, calorie control doesn't mean crash dieting or suddenly cutting off all calories. MD is done gradually.

The added benefit is that with fasting, you increase the HGH levels in your body that will fix all, or many of the problems you are having with your body, including your ability to burn off your fat.

So imagine combining calorie control with HGH! It's a **MAGIC DIET!**

WHEN IS THE BEST TIME TO EXERCISE?

Sports and exercise should be done in the morning or at the time of fasting before you put the food in.
 When I say food, I mean anything you put in your mouth and then you eat, with the exception of things that have no calories at all.

Many have said that you shouldn't exercise on empty stomach because your muscle will be consumed and you will not get stronger, or you will be sick, blah-blah-blah, yadda-yadda-yadda.
Let me think about that for a second NO!

Here is what the research says:

One of the key benefits of exercise and fasting is they both increase insulin sensitivity, and insulin sensitivity is an independent predictor of future mortality. But they work in different complementary ways.
Exercise for example, particularly short burst of HIT (High intensity training) depletes the glycogen stores in the muscles, while Intermittent Fasting (IF) depletes the glycogen stores in the liver.

The point is that if while in a state of fasting you exercise by lifting weights then your HGH will be increased!
Don't worry about the muscle loss that other people talk about.

Our bodies are smarter than that. It will take the reserves fat for your energy and it will burn your fat 4 times faster! It's possible that you will experience muscle loss if the fat in your body is minimal like that of a body builder, or below 7% of your total body weight.
What is your body fat percentage? The average is about 20%. At the time I wrote this my body fat percentage was somewhere between 9 and 12%.

Here is the best part! Because your HGH increases while you are fasting simple weight lifting will make your body gain muscle much faster.

"so many people have told me never to exercise on an empty stomach!"
Oh, is that so?

Why don't you try swimming on a full stomach! You like cramps? . . . I didn't think so!

Take a look at the cats and dogs in the street who are forced to hunt in the road for their meals.

They do it on an empty stomach and they eat only once a day if they are lucky. Compare them to pet cats and dogs that are fed 2 or three times a day at home. They quickly get fat and they die young.

Exercise before eating is very good!

And there might be benefits in doing that.

A lot of literature on this subject out there, with most of them reporting on studies about Muslims during Ramadan. They get a mix of positive and negative results but mostly negative.

But Ramadan month is very different from this kind of fasting. In the holy Ramadan fasting we are limiting food and water intake during the day. And you can dehydrate when you push yourself to do exercise.

In this type of fasting you still can drink water, so you will not dehydrate at all.

Second, because the eating and drinking is limited to pre-dawn and late afternoon hours, often you are sleep deprived. While in this type of fasting you can sleep.

Therefore, if you have enough sleep and you drink enough water and then exercise, you are fast will be different!!

The essence of MD part 2

Improved insulin sensitivity

The MD fast will increase your insulin sensitivity. The latest research found that this effect will be increased if you combine it with exercise.

At the end of the research, the subjects who fasted had a lower body weight (the only group that did not gain weight), had a better body glucose tolerance, and had increased insulin sensitivity.
 Furthermore, only with fasting did they significantly improve muscular adaptation to training.

Improved recovery from endurance training.

The subjects improved post-workout recovery, maintained body mass withoutfat, lowered fat mass, and maintained their performance.

Other studies demonstrated that fasting with endurance training may quickly re-activate the translation of muscle proteins derived from the fat of your body!

Improved Recovery from Weight Training

A study in 2009 found that subjects who lifted weights in a fasting state got "intramyocellular anabolic response."(indicator) Muscle growth in a fasting state doubled compared with those who eat before workout! (In the same group). In other words, fasting helps post-workout muscle growth.

Fasting does not directly give you super power, but it can maintain performance while enjoying the metabolic benefits, such as increased recovery, higher glycogen levels, better insulin sensitivity and enhanced muscle response to exercise.

The bottom line is that workouts in a fasting state will not kill you, will not eat your muscles, and may even increase the adaptation to exercise by forcing you to train in a state of "less optimal."

Consider this. At the time of slavery in the United States, African people suffered from a lack of food now have better genetics. How could their genes be bettercompared to us, since they wereslaves who ate less but worked harder?

Think about my words.

Remember!

The success of your training, whether it's lifting weights, walking, running, rowing, biking or climbing, doesn't entirely depend on your physical state, amount of glycogen in your muscle and liver, your tissues mobility, the structural size of your muscle cells, or the distribution of fiber in your muscle cells. These are all the factors that help to determine how strong you are.

Just as important is your mindset, your personal approach to fasting while training.

Suggestion: If you think you can not do this or if you limp, you'll limp. Have you ever heard stories of people getting chased by big dog and have no trouble jumping a high fence? It's the same with this! It's all in the **MIND SET**

I played a trick on my assistant. I felt bad about this, but it was so funny I couldn't resist.
 I asked him to exercise on an empty stomach.
He did and he had no strength to do the exercises.
He was limp and weak and had a very tough time getting through it.

The next day, while he was still in a state of fasting, I gave him a pill and told him that it was a new super supplement to increase blood sugar and energy to make him stronger.
An hour later, while still operating on an empty stomach he felt strong and was able to do the exercise with no problems.

 Want to know what was in the pill that I gave him?
 Tapioca!
I just went into my kitchen, filled up a small capsule and gave it to him.

Do you see what happened? Placebo pill! Placebo supplement!

And he felt strong!

YOU CAN WHEN YOU BELIEVE YOU CAN!

Believe it or not, it's true. Please! Try MD for one week and after that your strength for lifting weights will increase up to 75%. That's what happened to me! Before I ate and during my fasting hour, my lifting strength increased rapidly!

Never Did Cardio !!!

CARDIO? I DON'T

(This is my way and my thinking. You don't have to agree or argue with me because I've made up my mind and I'm not particularly concerned about it.)

A few days ago at the gym I saw an obese woman, her weight had to be more than 100 kilogram and she was running on the treadmill.

I asked myself how long will she be running on that?

If she pays attention to the machine which would tell her that she will start burning fat when her heart rate climbs over 122 bpm. I wondered just how long she would be able to sustain that.

Can Cardio (heart) exercise burn fat?
Actually, yes, it CAN, but only when you are there on the machine, and when you are running. Over time your body will grow accustomed to it and start burning muscle too.

On the other hand, weight lifting will damage your muscles and damaged muscle requires energy to repair and build. Consequently, it will, while you are fasting, burn your fat 2 X 24 hours long! WOW!

Do you want to burn fat

Forget cardio!! Or if you really feel the need to do cardio, do it after your weight lifting.

The following will invite controversy. Please read.

6 PACK WITHOUT SIT UPS

This will surprise a lot of people on the fact in the formation of abdominal muscles...

Forget sports or sit up or all the things you believe in all this time that will shape your stomach...

They are all bullshit...

Did you know that a lot of people at the gym who have 6 packs will lie to you if you ask them how they got that way?

Who doesn't want to have nicely shaped stomach? Both men and women?

This is a dream of men of all ages and in the imagination of women about all the men. Yes it is, **please, stop lying to yourself by saying you don't.**

Unfortunately this is the most difficult part of your body to form. You can build your arm muscles or your chest or any other part of your body with relative ease. But forming stomach muscle? Now that's another story!

I was born with very bad genes. I have an endomorph body type. This means I was born fat. I will live fat, and I will die fat. I was very jealous of those who were born with what I felt were better genes.

You know them, the slim waisted, broad shouldered, well formed mesomorphs. I was so jealous! I hated them!

No, I actually envied them.

Every time I exercised or went to the gym I saw younger people with nicer bodies, I started blaming my genes.
 I thought that maybe with aggressive exercises like sit ups or cardio mile on the treadmill that I would form my stomach muscles.
I did sit ups, 100 repetitions a day. I got results from this, but not what I was looking for.
I discovered a hard cold reality. SIT UP ONLY MAKE YOUR STOMACH LARGER! Imagine a balloon.
Whatever you fill in a balloon whether water, air or anything, it will make the balloon become bigger and bigger. It's the same with your stomach. If you fill it with muscle, it will get bigger.

Never Did Sit Ups Again !!!

So I STOPPED and I NEVER DID SIT UPS AGAIN! Then and only then is when I built my 6 abs for the first time at age 37.

So how? You ask me.

1. Forget stomach exercises like sit ups or cardio or the treadmill.

2. Forget infomercial products such as massage belts or whatsoever they advertise that promises to make you slimmer. All they do is

eliminate water. Your fat will not disappear with vibration. Come on! You're smarter than that!

3. Forget slimming pills, slimming tea or slimming cream and all the empty promises. (Most of them only make you sick). There are no magic pills! This is why all diet products have a small notification which says: must be accompanied with regular diet and exercise. Oh! Come on! Don't you think that with regular diet and exercise you have no need for a pill?

4. Forget about buying food with NO FAT or ZERO FAT or LOW FAT labels! The fact is we need it, and fat is not our enemy in food! The right kind of fat can actually make you slim!

So how can I get a well defined six pack?

1. The theory is easy to understand. Everybody, both men and women have muscle in their stomach. Without it, you cannot sit, or stand up. Try to imagine having a stomach without muscle. Everybody has a six pack. The only thing you need to do is remove the fat that covers it. YOU CAN'T DO THAT WITH SIT UPS! 1,000,000,000 sit ups a day will make your stomach larger!

2. Stomach building starts with the mouth, not at the gym!
There are no exercises that can give your stomach 6 packs. You can use exercise to tighten it if you already have six packs, but if not it will thicken the layers of fat covering it

and it will make you look fatter! Do you want to do sit ups?
WAIT UNTIL YOUR BODY FAT RATIO IS UNDER 15%.

3. How many times do I have to do sit ups or do other stomach exercises? NO NEED! You already train your muscles every day by sitting down, standing up, and even walking. This is a kind of training you do every day without realizing it. So, forget about training your stomach muscles. You will only get cramps, or your stomach gets fatter. Wait until your body fat ratio is under at least 15%. That's when you can do sit ups to thicken up your stomach muscle if you feel that it's necessary. As for me, I can count the amount of sit ups I do in a year on my fingers.

The only way to get six packs is to lower your BODY FAT! Yes! BODY! Not stomach fat! Lower it down to 12%.
Don't do it with CARDIO! Cardio means just that, cardio. Cardio means HEART, not fat elimination.

Weight lifting will burn your fat in 2 X 24 hours even while you sleep. (Weight lifting VS cardio is another story altogether.)
A lot of people think that weight lifting will make them become bigger.
DO YOU THINK THAT IT'S EASY TO BECOME BIG and MUSCULAR? Yes, weight lifting will make you big (FAT) because after weight lifting you EAT A LOT!

And a lot of women are afraid to have big

muscles. WOMEN WILL NOT BECOME BIG BY WEIGHT LIFTING! They simply don't have as much testosterone as men. **The muscular woman you see on magazine covers is a result of steroid injections! You will not become big if you follow my MD diet! Excuses like this are only to cover up for laziness!**

4. Food, yes, food and only food; the amount of calories that you take into your body is what matters. If you burn 1500 calories in a day, but eat 2000 calories (there are ways of counting this) even if it's healthy, clean food or only an apple and a banana, YOU WILL STORE FAT EVERY DAY! If you eat fatty unhealthy food but the total amount is below the amount of calories you burn in a day, you will use up your fat reserves. Whether or not it's clean food or fatty food it is no problem as long as you control the calories. (But, by following MD, you can forget all of this because it will be enough.

5. Stop taking pictures of your food and posting it in social media with PRIDE.
Why do you do this? Do you want to show people that you are a piggy, or what? Now, on the other hand if they are hobby food pictures, that's not a problem. But do us all a favor and list the calorie content along with it. Believe it or not, this will make you lose weight faster. There is research that says that people who put food photos up with the caloric content written below it have significant weight loss. WOW!

THE MONK'S SECRET Breathing ON MUSCLE BUILDING.

I have my own method of weight lifting which is different than that of the common way, (another of the monk's secrets.)
It makes muscle development 4 times more effective than the usual exercise routines. I spend 15 to 20 minutes at the gym 3 times a week and I don't bother with cardio or sit ups.

Maybe you will ask if the ancient Shaolin is muscular?

The simple answer is that some of them are and some of them are not. It all really depends on their training. Some are trained in Kungfu and some are trained for some other martial art.

One example is that the Kungfu tiger stance requires certain muscles to execute. Consequently they are trained to build certain muscle groups.

 Whereas the crane moves don't require muscle so much as they require speed and so they are trained to be fast with smaller mature muscles.

Breathing Techniques

Breathing Increases Muscle! Breathing is the oxygenation process to all of the cells in your body. With the supply of oxygen to the brain, this increases the muscles in your body.

5 minute abdominal breathing technique before exercise.

Do you know the difference between breathing from your abdomen and breathing with your chest? Watch a newborn baby or a young child sleeping quietly in their beds. It's their stomach that enlarges and then shrinks.

It's because they breathe naturally with the stomach and not with the chest. As time goes on and we age, we change out breathing patterns from the stomach to the chest. It could be that because we are ashamed of the size of our stomachs, and so without realizing it we switch to

breathing with our chest and pull in our stomach. YOU ARE DOING IT RIGHT NOW!

Deep breathing provides oxygen to your cells of your body, which helps you absorb nutrients. It also stimulates your lymphatic system to get rid of toxins. If you are breathing shallow, also known as chest breathing, your cells receive less nutrient and your lymph system may be slower. Both of these factors will cause you to gain weight.

The monks as a matter of regular habit do light meditation before they exercise.

THE MONK'S SECRET : Here is How

THE MONK'S SECRET ON MUSCLE BUILDING.

Before you do your workout:

Close your eyes, inhale through your abdomen and not
your chest slowly, make one inhalation 20 seconds,
hold your breath for 10 seconds then exhale slowly, so
for one inhale and exhale you need about 1 minute!

Do this 5 minutes before you lifting weights at gym.
You will notice that this makes a difference.

On workout:

Try this now and inhale deep then hold and tighten
your body muscle. Hold that for a few moments. Feel
the sensation of hardness. Now, slowly, while your
muscle is still tight, exhale.
What happens? You muscle relaxes.

This is what the monks do when they are lifting
weights.

Inhale, lift up your weights for 3 seconds with slow
motion, hold your load for few seconds then release
your breath and slowly lower it down.

*Proper Breathing assists in Weight Control. If you are
overweight, the extra oxygen burns up the excess fat
more efficiently. If you are underweight, the extra
oxygen feeds the starving tissues and glands.*

Wing Chun Stroke

**Wing Chun Stroke and other theories of weight
lifting**

As a practitioner of Wing Chun and as an international instructor, I use this self-defense theory in weight training.

Most gymnasium members lift their weights with a pattern of repetition with a light load, such as 5 kilograms of weight with 20 repetitions. This is identical to a construction worker lifting sand with the same weight repeated many times until your body memorizes the pattern.
Look at the body of a construction worker. Dry, dry porters. If that's what you want, by all means, keep doing it.

I will let you slap my face three times as hard as you can, if you will let me punch you in the face only once but really hard. Want to do that?

Which one do you think is more painful? Which one will have the more severe impact?

The concept of muscle building is to "damage" our muscles and build them up again while resting. This is why I spend only 15 to 20 minutes at the gym, because I don't need a long arduous, repetitious workout to make my muscle stronger.
This could be contrary to the concept of a professional body builder, but then, I'm not a professional body builder.

How do I do it?

I start with the body builder's concept. I divide my muscles into 2 main groups; big and small muscles. Big muscles include the chest, back, shoulders and legs. The small muscles are the arms; biceps and triceps.

The procedure is that I train 1 big muscle and 1 small muscle a day, skip one day, (keep doing M7W) and continue by doing the other muscles the next day.

1. Chest and triceps

2. MD 7 minutes workout (I will explain this later)

3. Back and biceps

4. M7W

5. Shoulder and triceps

6. M7W

7. Leg

This fits with 7 days a week.

And because it only takes less than 30 minutes then there is no excuse for not having the time. I will tell you to do your exercise before you have eaten, but if that's not possible, you car still do it any time.

How to do the training?

You can google for the instructions on how to train muscles. You can ask an instructor at your local gym or contact us and talk to an MD instructor, but the problem is knowing how much weight you should lift. You don't want to emaciate your body like a porter.

I just use 6 repetitions.

(6 times lifting multiple 3 times in one tool, one muscle use 3 tools or 3 different games)

For example:

Chest with the bench press 6X3 then butterfly press 6X3 and the last maybe upper chest 6X3.

Why only 6 times? That's your question, yes because I only can do 6 times..I will look for a very heavy burden which I only can lift it most 6 times, sometimes only 4 times.

Every 6 repetition I take 30 seconds rest then lift again to start the second 6 repetition and so on. Every time I change tool I only rest for 1 minutes... this will damage our muscle.

I always lift the heaviest weight that I can. If I find that I can lift it 8 more times then it's too light. Is there more damage done with three hard slaps or if you punch only once? That's the idea.

In this way I only spent a short time for my muscle development.

M7W : What is ?

What is M7W or MD 7 minutes workout?

This is not a new concept so the sport practitioners do not need to fuss about it and claim that I copied the old way, but is rarely used by people to train their bodies.

 It only takes 7 minutes of your time a day and you can do that over and over again when you have extra time on that day. So there is no reason to not do this if it takes only 7 minutes.

This training is commonly known as High intensive training.

M7W training is very useful to burn fat and build your muscles at the same time. Intensive exercise with fast repetition will actually boost your HGH level. Imagine how doing this will boost your HGH levels if this is done while you are fasting.

In addition, this training is done without the need for tools, weights or equipment so you can do it anywhere.

The advantage of M7W is:

1. To strengthen all parts of your muscle and promote HGH.

2. No need for weights, tools or equipment, so you can to it anywhere.

3. Burn off excess fat faster in a shorter period of time compared to spending time on your cardio machine or aerobic training.

4. You can do it repeatedly again and again in the same day.

M7W can be a faster and efficient way to lose excess weight and our body fat. This type of resistance training makes a significant contribution to the amount of fat burned during exercise.

When we do this resistance training we use some big muscles with just a little rest between sets, it results in aerobic and metabolic benefits simultaneously.

Research into this has found that the metabolic benefit can be present up to 72 hours after the workout is completed!

Here is how:

Following is an example of M7W program. All exercises can be done with your own body weight and can be implemented anywhere; your home, your office, your hotel room or anywhere that is convenient to you.

This exercise is performed for 30 seconds of movement with a 10 second transition time (break) between different styles of exercise. The total time for the whole exercise is about 7 minutes. The series can be repeated 2 to 3 times.

M7W : Practice

MD 7 Minutes Workout : Practice

1. Jumping jacks 30 seconds (to train the all muscles).

2. Sitting position to hold body on the wall 30 seconds (lower muscle).

3. Push-up 30 seconds (upper muscles).

4. Stomach crunches 30 seconds (abdominal training here is used for intensity of your middle muscles).

5. Up and down chair or stairs (whole muscles) 30 seconds.

6. Squat 30 seconds (lower muscles).

7. Triceps with chair (upper muscles) 30 seconds.

8. Plank (muscles balance) 30 seconds.

9. High knee movement / running in place (cardio) 30 seconds.

10. Lunge (lower muscles) 30 seconds.

11. Push-up and rotation (upper muscles) 30 seconds.

12. Side plank (whole body) 30 seconds.

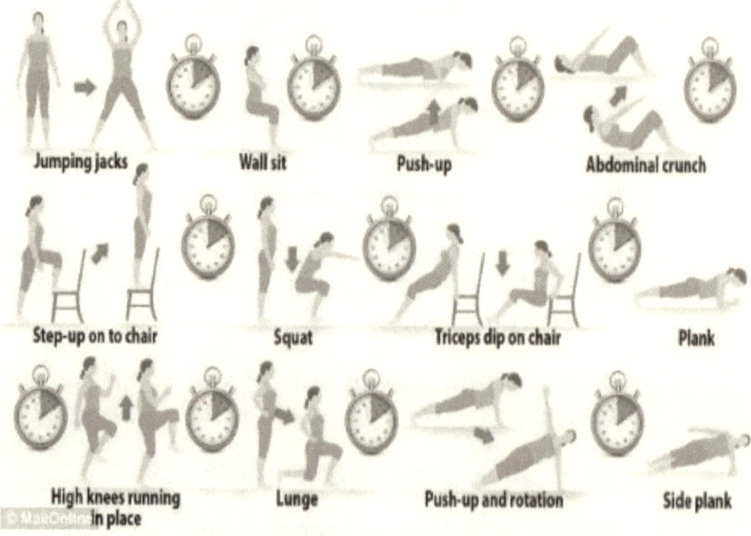

Each training exercise is interspersed with only 10 seconds of rest in between.

The easiest way to keep pace is to use the timer in your mobile phone .

M7W can be an efficient way of doing exercises to help lower body fat, improve insulin sensitivity and improve your heart and increase muscle mass.

Using your own body weight for M7W makes exercising practical and more accessible because you are already athletic enough to lift it.

For those who have maintained that you have no time, or money for exercise, now there is no excuse, and the benefits of these kinds of exercises are the same and even better for your health and fitness, compared to other forms.

IF YOU ARE NOT PHYSICALLY ABLE, DO NOT FORCE YOURSELF TO DO M7W. START SLOWLY AND GRADUALLY INCREASE THE EFFORT UNTIL YOUR BODY GROWS ACCUSTOMED TO IT.

I am certain there will be many agreements and disagreements about this writing and I'm also certain that you have in mind lots of questions that I am unable to answer here.
Keep in mind that all of this belongs to a theory that I have practiced on my own and have enjoyed much success along with many of my friends.
So, the ball is in your court. You can do as you please, but I will keep telling you that there is nothing wrong with this theory of diet and exercise.

Lately, a lot of people have been comparing my therory with other forms of bodybuilding and nutrition attached to famous names. This is just silly. They are all great, but in their own field which cannot be compared to mine.

For me, MD is not a fad diet to be done periodically. It's a way of life, and I wish that you all agreed with it. If not, it's your choice and I wish you good luck in whatever you do.
One final thought:

I build up my body so that I can play with my son and keep up with him. He runs over here, over there and every which way and because I'm in better condition, I can keep up with him.

I do have a genetic predisposition towards cancer, and I'm doing my best to fight it. (
But, you never know what will happen.

FAQ : Is This Just a Trend?

Is This Just a Trend?

I have been asked repeatedly if this is merely a fad diet that will be popular for a short time but then quickly end.

This is an easy question to answer.
 For some, a diet is merely a temporary trend; just a fad for them to do until they grow tired of it and move on to find something else.
For others, it becomes a permanent lifestyle. This is why that for me, it's my way of life.

As I write this it is already my daily lifestyle. There are times I have done MD for the entire week with a 24 hour fast and I consider it good clean fun.

MD is much easier to adopt as a lifestyle than other diets which prohibit you from eating any tasty food; the kind that you love to eat. It is a human tendency to have a lust of the mouth that will cause you to break other kinds of diets and force you to start all over again.

 I've asked people again and again. "Would you rather eat a lot of bland and tasteless food, or would you rather eat anything you like in modest amounts in a limited time?" The overwhelming majority consistently chooses the second option. So my answer is that this will not be a fad or a trend. It will become a way of life.

FAQ : Skipping Breakfast???

Skipping Breakfast?

Those who disagree with me always attack my theory on the issue of breakfast. One media outlet claimed that skipping breakfast leads to heart disease. Let's read again what issues really cause heart disease.

They claim that by not eating a good breakfast will prompt us to eat too much at lunch time, and this will cause us to get fatter. I strongly take issue with this idea because that research is biased and doesn't take into account other factors.

There are valid studies that have concluded that eating or not eating breakfast has nothing to do with how much we eat at lunch time.

So who are you going to believe? Greedy overeating is a mindset. If your goal is to eat blindly, with reckless abandon, what's the point of dieting at all? If you have no dietary goals perhaps it does in fact increase your desire to eat more at lunch.

My breakfast time now is 4:00 Pm and so far I am very fit and I don't feel any hunger in my activity. It's all in your mind. If you don't want to over eat, you won't and you can beat your appetite.

FAQ : Junk Food vs Good Food???

Junk Food vs Good Food?

I never said that healthy food isn't good. What I said was that according to how I feel about it, "healthy" food is usually tasteless. Let's just examine the facts.

 If healthy food is tasty then people will eat it without the need to ask them to and as a result, everybody would be healthy.

Is that right? Well, unfortunately this is simply not true. It's a shame, but we enjoy unhealthy food more than with healthy food.

So, if you can eat healthy food while you're doing MD that's really great. As for myself, I mix it. Sometimes I eat healthy food and sometimes I want to enjoy my food . . . sometimes, not always.

FAQ : Its not Healthy???

Its not Healthy

Once again I have never said that eating dirty food will make you healthy.

NO, I never said that at all. Some media outlets have said that because MD encourages you to eat "dirty and gross food" it will cause you to pile up the diseases for later times.

 To me this is hilarious. What's their definition of "dirty or gross food?" Is it Fried rice? Fried chicken? Lemak rice? Let me shed some light on it.

What is obesity? Obesity is a form of disease. 75% of all heart disease is caused by obesity. How about if we take care of the problems one by one and do the most important ones first? My highest priority target is to remove obesity from our bodies.

If our body shape is good, our fat is decreased. Consequently the likelihood of illness will also decrease. This is common sense and easy to understand is it not?

Do you want to eat healthy food while you are doing MD? Please do so.

Good for you and I support that. I want for you to deal with the problems one by one, starting with your weight.

When you have achieved your ideal weight, then you will appreciate your health a lot more. As far as my opinion goes, any food that you eat, as long as your body burns it off it will have no deleterious effect on you.

all, we don't eat poison. Who says that eating fat is not healthy, who says that goat meat isn't healthy?

For sure many people have their own peculiar allergies, so if you have high blood pressure you know that goat meat is definitely unhealthy for you, if you have low blood pressure then you know that it's good for you.

So it's not a FIXED formula for everyone. And another thing, who says that high cholesterol is unhealthy? I will talk about this later.

Exercise with empty stomach???

"NO! I Can't do that!" Says who? These are slacker words!
 It has been proven that HGH increases when you are fasting, but also your energy and strength increases. If you are lazy, well, that's a real problem isn't it?
 My energy is doubled when I exercise on an empty stomach.

Bulking VS Sculpting

Many asked me if MD can be used for Bulking up; increasing muscle mass?
The answer is YES, but with MD, according to me you avoid the mistakes that a bodybuilder makes.

They bulk up with heavy lifting and consuming 3-4000 calories a day with the hope that a bigger body means heavier lifting.
They get bigger muscles and then later on they will diet like crazy to remove the fat that it creates.

Yes, it works but remember that they are taking their life into their hands. With bulking your level of fat increases more rapidly compared to the increase of their muscle.
 There are a lot of wannabe bodybuilders who bulked up and stayed that way because they were too tired, or too lazy to do the necessary sculpting.

This is why I think that bulking up in MD is superior. First, can MD increase your body weight? Yes, it can. Don't forget that the weight that you want to add is muscle, not fat.

This is how you proceed: First, you measure the percentage of your body fat. There are plenty of tools around that can help you do this.
You can find weight scales at the gym or at your local drug store that will measure your body fat ratio.

The most well known system for this is called OMRON. Make sure your fat level is below 15%. remember the term "little fat man" and "little fat girl" where you think you are skinny but your body only contains fat and it's a lot) so if your fat level is still 15% or above, it is better to not think about fattening your body.

Well, let's see how to make your muscles bigger using MD. The way is in is through your eating window, 4 hours or 6 hours, eat food with that has a higher calorie content than your burned calories, so if you burn calories (average 1500 for women and 2000 for men) then add more calories eg 500 calories a day (2000 for women or 3000 men) and add to it more weight lifting exercises.

 While you're doing this, measure your fat percentage every week. If your fat ratio is above 15%, reduce the caloric intake! Maintain a 15% ratio in your body and it will be easy to reduce your fat level.

 If the fat level rises above 15% it will be more difficult. Don't listen to the advice of a bodybuilder if you don't want to become bodybuilder.

I'm not referring to all bodybuilders, because a lot of them are right in what they say and are good at giving advice. I really like Mr.Arnold Schwarzenegger. I think he is good at helping people and many of them are actually good.

I hope that if there are any bodybuilders reading this, you could become a good adviser to us, non bodybuilders without making us offers for steroids or drugs.

Women and Muscle.

"I am a woman and I'm afraid becoming muscular." This is a concern that is often expressed to me. I always tell them not to worry about it.

 It's hard to build muscles, even if you are a guy so relax.

You will not become muscular like a man unless you deliberately inject your body with steroids.
Most female professional body builders use drugs or steroids.

Women have only a small amount of testosterone and they can't build muscle like men can.
If your weight becomes heavy without being bulky you will be sexy and the better shape you will be in.
 You won't become bulky like a man.

Facts!!! How Good Having : Surprise

High Cholesterol is ON YOUR MD!

Blaming cholesterol for causing your heart disease is like blame the firefighters if your house burns down.

We need to talk about this.

At the time you are fasting, your cholesterol level will rise rapidly. Would that terrify you?

Research Cardiologist at the Intermountain Medical Center Heart Institute in Murray, Utah, in one of their research by Dr. Benjamin D. Home said that LDL will rise about 14% and HDL about 6% when fasting. This is not a bad thing.

Fasting stresses our body from within and our body responds by releasing more cholesterol. You are using fat as your fuel and not sugars, and this is a good way to avoid diabetes.

The article below is based on the summary and on research performed by Jonny Bowden PhD., C.N.S., Stephen Sinatra M.D., F.A.C.C and many other doctors who want to open our eyes to the truth about cholesterol and the lies about it.

This is my story:

In 2007, my dad was hospitalized. He told me it was because of an ulcer. On December 30th, two days after my birthday he was admitted to the hospital. On January 1st he died. The doctor's diagnosis was that he'd died of HEART failure along with some complications.

Sadly, I had to accept it.

When I asked him what had caused it, the doctor said that it was a result of high cholesterol and that it was inevitable that it would have happened eventually. "How high doctor?" I asked...

"Hmmm," he said. "It was above 200."

He sounded like he wasn't certain, and by the manner of his speech I wondered if he even remembered.

This brought panic to my heart and I feel stupid for being silent and not pressing him for the truth. Instead I was silent.

In my heart I still remember what I was thinking at the moment.

"What really happened?"

- Most of his life my dad kept himself on a strict diet.

- My dad exercised almost every morning.

- My dad didn't smoke and he didn't drink alcohol.

Cholesterol????

From where? Is it really true that CHOLESTEROL killed him?

Ladies and gentlemen, in 2010 I went in and had my cholesterol levels checked and discovered that they had reached 500.

Can you imagine how scared that made me? What do you think my doctor told me? He said that it was hereditary and I would have to take a drug called "L" for the rest of my life. So, for the rest of my life, I took

"L", that is until 2012.

That was when I began to experiment with my MD theory and discovered that a human can change/alter their genetic factor. So I figure that if I can alter my genetic tendency from obesity and go from 100 kilograms down to 73 kilograms with good muscle mass I can also alter my natural tendency towards high cholesterol. It should work that way, right?

I began a search for the real answers, and I kept on searching until I found a very surprising answer. This will surprise you too. This will open the eyes of most doctors and make them realize that they need to learn something all over again.

And, what truth is this?

Read carefully, this will come as a surprise.

Facts!!! How Good Having : DEATH

CHOLESTEROL DOES NOT LEAD TO DEATH BY HEART DISEASE

Yes, you read it right.

THE HIGHER YOUR CHOLESTEROL LEVEL THE LONGER YOU LIVE.

Wow! Yes, you read that correctly too.

ANTI CHOLESTEROL DRUGS WILL SLOWLY KILL YOU!

This claim might seem a bit outrageous but the truth is in the proof. We'll get to that later.
You can jump out of your seat and run to tell your parents, or perhaps keep reading and hear me out on this.

WHAT IS CHOLESTEROL?

Cholesterol is a type of oil that is made in your liver and is an absolute necessity for the individual cells of your body.

Cholesterol is needed for the manufacturing of vitamin D and for hormones such as estrogen, progesterone and testosterone. There are two fundamental types of cholesterol; HDL and LDL. Almost all the present knowledge about cholesterol is out of date.

Facts!!! How Good Having : HDL

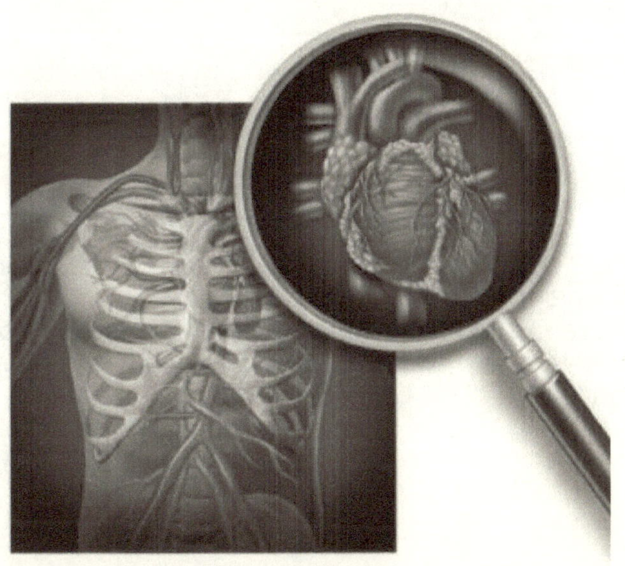

High-density lipoproteins (HDL)

Old information about HDL:

HDL is considered to be the healthy type of cholesterol which eliminates bad cholesterol or LDL. Most hoped that they could bring their HDL up to as high as possible. It was considered to be very good if it reached above 60mg/dl or more..

If you maintain your body weight, stay on a good diet,
exercise regularly and etc. it was considered a factor
in increasing the HDL levels in the body.

Now there are new studies with a better understanding
of HDL. HDL has more influence on genetic tendencies
compared to LDL.
Research in 2011, at the National Institutes of Health
has revealed that increased HDL will not help to
reduce the risk of heart attack or stroke at all. It is
now known that HDL is divided into two types.

HDL-2 is large and soft, it floats and is good.

HDL-3 is small and hard and can cause blockage in
your bloodstream.
So even HDL, which was considered a good type of
cholesterol turned out to be not as good as previously
thought.

Facts!!! How Good Having : LDL

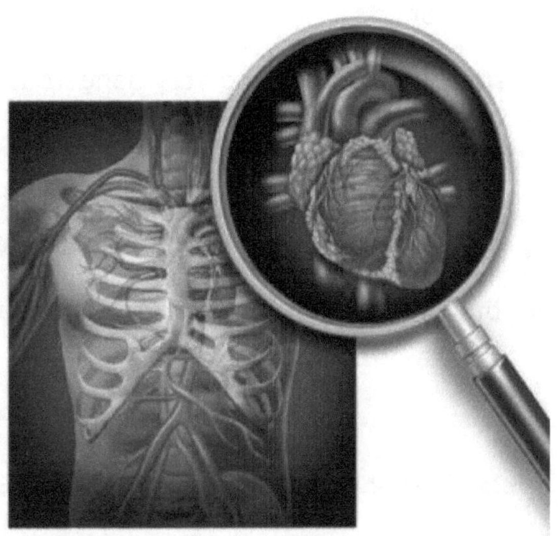

Low-Density Lipoprotein (LDL)

Old understanding:

LDL is the bad type of cholesterol which must be lowered at all costs because it interferes with the blood running through the veins.
The ideal target for blood content for LDL is 100mg/dl or lower.
 Eating food with high fat content and a lack of exercise can make your LDL levels higher, and this can kill you.

The new understanding of LDL:

It turns out that LDL is not completely bad because there are 2 kinds of LDL found in the human body.

LDL-A is the large, soft floating type and as long as there is no oxidation from the outside (free radicals) then you are safe.

LDL-B is small hard, sticky and very dangerous. This is the type of cholesterol that forms plaque inside your arteries, causes blockages and can kill you.

Interestingly in the present time you can check for both types of this cholesterol through a laboratory. Unfortunately, most doctors will not ask you to have it checked, but simply offer you drugs to control it!

Facts!!! How Good Having : CHOLESTEROL

CHOLESTEROL CHECK UP

WHAT USUALLY HAPPENS:

The doctor takes a blood sample and sends it to a lab. The lab sends back the results. If the total amount of your LDL and HDL levels are high, the doctor writes you a prescription for drugs.

THE WAY IT SHOULD BE DONE:

When you are in for a cholesterol check, request an in-depth detailed examination.
Find out how much LDL type A and type B that you have, but more important, find out how much Lp(a) you have so you know how much danger you are in.

Lp(a) is a low-density lipoprotein type, or LDL ("bad")
cholesterol.
 A high level of Lp(a) can cause plaque to form in your
arteries.
 This type of cholesterol buildup restricts the flow of
blood through your arteries.
A high level of Lp(a) can be an indicator of cholesterol-
related disease, such as coronary artery disease.

Research has found it to be an independent risk factor
for heart disease, even though it is not been defined
exactly how the information can be used in routine
treatment.

 The point is that knowing only your LDL isn't enough
to say whether or not you are at risk to get heart
disease.

SETTING UP THE RIGHT DIET

ANTIQUATED THINKING

Eat no more than 300 mg of cholesterol in one day.
Your total food intake for the day should never exceed
10% in order to reduce your cholesterol levels.

MORE UP TO DATE THINKING

According to research done in the Framingham Heart
Study, the amount of cholesterol in the blood of
people who consumed food containing high or low
cholesterol content had no effect on the amount of
cholesterol in their blood.

Every person is unique and most people are unaffected
by the amount of cholesterol they consume in their
food.

Even when there is a noticeable effect, the difference was in the HDL (good) and not in the LDL. (bad) To this day, there is no evidence that fatty foods influences heart disease except for those foods that contain TRANS FAT, SUGAR AND OMEGA 6.

This is the history:

When The National Cholesterol Education in 2004 suggested a reduction of cholesterol, 8 out of 9 people at that agency were representing cholesterol drug companies.

Again, I have to remind you that if you read my writing, or if you get advice from your doctor you should always be critical and check the sources of their information. Google is your best resource to find the truth.

This controversy first began when a Russian scientists provided a number of experiments on rabbits by feeding them high cholesterol food and then dissected them to see what they would find. What they found was a great deal of plaque in the arteries identical to the plaque in the arteries in patients who had died of heart failure.

What they failed to point out is that a rabbit is a strict herbivore, and that it had been fed with high cholesterol food. What's wrong with this picture?

When the same experiments were conducted on mice or monkeys, the results were quite different. Even the key researchers declared in 1997 that there was no connection between the cholesterol in the food and the cholesterol in the body, unless of course you happen to be a rabbit.

John Yudkin a doctor from the British University of London said that "according to the latest data, most heart disease is caused by SUGAR."

Facts!!! How Good Having : Phenomenon 1

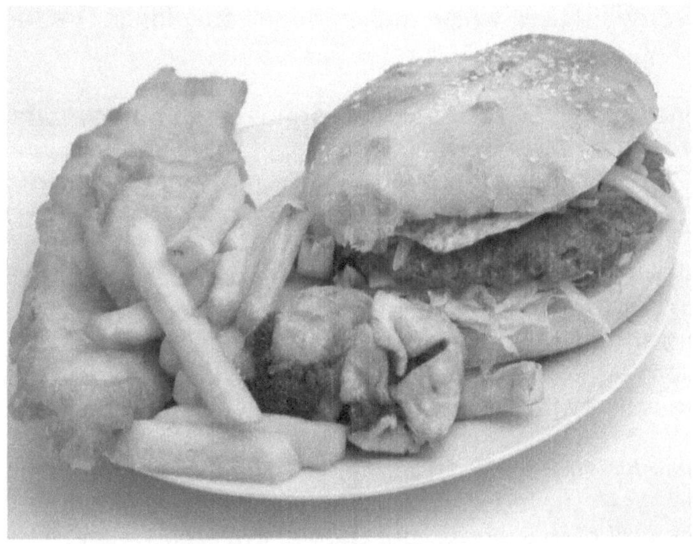

The phenomenon of food without cholesterol 1

After almost everybody began believing that cholesterol was dangerous then food products further promoted the idea by capitalizing on the fear.
They began aggressively promoting food with "low fat, low cholesterol" labels and they replaced the fat and cholesterol content with sugar and carbohydrates for flavor.

This was more dangerous compared to the fat itself because sugar becomes fat when it's processced in our bodies.

Saturated fat vs. Trans fat :

The saturated fats that food contains is natural. Trans fat is man-made fat which is created in a process by adding hydrogen into vegetable oil. This is called hydrogenation, which makes the oil stay longer in the body.

One kind of Trans fat is margarine. Lately, many food products advertise that Trans fats are healthier when in fact it has been proven that Trans fats are related to heart disease.

This is why, when there are more products in the U.S. that claim to be low fat, there is more obesity in the U.S. than anywhere else. The consequence is that the more afraid we are of destroying our bodies, the more we will eat food that we think is safe for us.

Dwight Lundell, M.D., author of "The Cure for Heart Disease", stated that "all this time we were catching the bull by the horns, but then discovered we were catching the wrong bull!"

De Lorgeril the chief of Lyon Diet Heart research, "we can summarize it with one sentence. Cholesterol is harmless".

THE ACTUAL CAUSE OF HEART DISEASE

The answer is inflammation.

The first type of inflammation is acute inflammation.

Whether it's from an itchy rash, a knife cut, or from a bruise you can feel the pain. It's called acute inflammation.

The kind of inflammation we are concerned with is chronic inflamation.
Chronic inflammation can kill us.

Chronic inflammation causes diseases like Alzheimers, cancer, diabetes, liver and especially heart disease.

The inflammation spreads so that is why you will often hear that someone died from the complications of the disease.
Inflammation in one place can be spread every where including up into your heart.

Facts!!! How Good Having : Phenomenon 2

The phenomenon of food without cholesterol 2

So the causes of death by heart attack are:

- Oxidation such as smoking etc

- Inflammation

- Stress

- Sugar and carbohydrates

Here is something strange. Cholesterol in our body is used to fight toxins, and that's why it is discovered in the arteries involved with inflammation. Blaming cholesterol as the killer is a lot like blaming a firefighter for burning your house down.

EXCESSIVELY low cholesterol is very dangerous!

Cholesterol is a source of vitamin D, sex hormones and are vehicles that deliver toxin fighters.

The latest research says that lower cholesterol levels can cause death from cancer, suicide and accidents.

Suicide?!

You need cholesterol to repair cells in your brain. If your cholesterol level is lower than 160 it can cause depression. And what happens sometimes to people when they get depressed? Think about that.

Therefore, the cholesterol lowering drugs can be dangerous. In his book "The Great Cholesterol Myth" Dr. Johnny Bowden said that drugs such as Lipitor is a "memory thief" that causes depression and memory loss.

Cholesterol is also used to help fight infections in our bodies. When we have an infection the total cholesterol level goes up, but your HDL will go down because it's being used to fight off the infection. When we are fasting we are detoxifying our bodies and this is why our HDL level decreases.

Remember again that LDL or bad cholesterol (which we think is evil) is divided into 2 types, lipo a and lipo b...unfortunately the doctor usually didn't care and doesn't ask you to check which one is higher and directly gives you drug to lower your cholesterol level. Next time, don't forget to ask your doctor to check your LDL in more detail, which LDL and find out which one is higher.

Dr. Beverly Teter from the University of Maryland said that cholesterol in blood tissues and arteries are there to treat inflammation. When death occurs and a higher level of cholesterol is discovered and then blamed as the cause is a big mistake!" Unfortunately many doctors don't want to acknowledge this and learn this new information.

What do you think happens when you purposely lower your cholesterol levels?

 People with high cholesterol live longer than those with a lower cholesterol level.
Don't worry about fatty or cholesterol rich foods. Stay away from trans fat and omega 6 foods such as pure vegetable oil.
Take omega 3 which is good for your body. Replace margarine with butter. Reduce sugar and carbohydrates.
Remember that from ancient times, heart disease increased when mankind entered the time of cultivation. More people began to eat sugar and carbohydrates such as rice, bread, and doughnuts with sugar, for example.

TRANS FATS and SUGAR have also been connected to autism. That could very well be why there are more people with autism in these times. EVERY MORNING YOU MAKE BREAKFAST FOR YOUR CHILDREN WHICH CONTAINS . . .

Why, after all this time have the researchers been so wrong about cholesterol being the cause of all this trouble?
Simple. They observed that there are firefighters in every fire, and made the assumption that they were the cause of it.

THERE IS A BETTER WAY TO PREDICT YOUR RISK OF HEART PROBLEMS WITH YOUR CHOLESTEROL LEVEL:

Look at you triglycerides and HDL levels. Make a comparison between those two.
For example if your triglyceride is 150 mg/dl and your HDL is 50mg/dl then the ratio between them is 150/50 or simply, 3.

If your triglyceride 100 and your HDL 50 so the ratio is 100/50 and the result is 2.
This is a better indication as to whether or not you are at risk of heart attack because of cholesterol.

A Harvard study for The American Heart Association said that if you have a high ratio your risk of heart attack is 16 times greater.

So if your comparison ratio is 2 or 3 you are still safe, if the ratio is 4 or 5 you have to be careful.

Facts!!! How Good Having : Effects

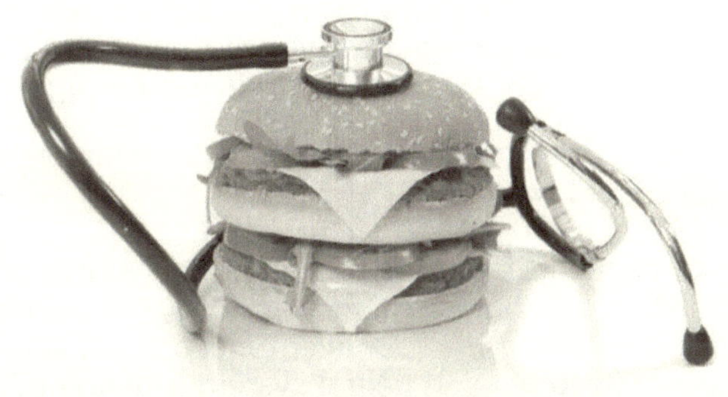

STATIN AND CHOLESTEROL DRUGS EFFECTS

People between the age of 40 to 45 are 50 percent more likely to develop Alzheimer's with high cholesterol than with low cholesterol.

That sounds pretty scary right?

This is an interesting statement from Robert Scott Bell D.A.Hom:

"For several generations we have grown to accept the "fact" that bad cholesterol or LDL should remain low no matter how much it costs. It doesn't seem matter that it is important for the health of your brain and nervous systems function. As long as the drug companies can keep us in fear of fat they will have us as loyal customers for as long as we live."

The research says that high cholesterol

**levels in your middle age will cause Alzheimer's when you reach old age.
Why? Let's think carefully about this. What happens to most adults diagnosed with "high" cholesterol in their middle age?**

They're doctors prescribe statin drugs to lower their cholesterol levels.

What happens if you are forced to reduce the availability of cholesterol for your body? The endocrine functions will suffer. Your liver functions will slow down. Your brain and neural system is degraded. In other words, statin drugs are what actually trigger brain diseases such as Alzheimer's.

So it is clear that what makes you suffer from ALZHEIMER'S, are cholesterol drugs such as Lipitor. Keep in mind that the profits from Lipitor are in excess of 30 million USD per year.

So, if you want to be senile, by all means, take it.

"CHOLESTEROL DOES NOT CAUSE HEART DISEASE!"

"Cholesterol is a friend that can make us healthier and help us to stay young. The reality is that a world drug syndicate is actually taking advantage of us." -Robert Scott

Dr. Bob DeMaria (The drugless doctor) said that the most evil drugs that are sold freely and most profitable for pharmacy is statin, such as Lipitor.

This causes liver damage, Alzheimer's, Parkinson's, stroke and so many other diseases.

Do you want to reduce your cholesterol level?
 Eat a juicy red apple once a day. That's it. But remember cholesterol is not what causes you to have a heart attack and die.

Facts!!! How Good Having : Controversy

This is going to cause some extraordinary controversy.

Some doctors are not going to like this.
 When I entered a tweet in twitter .com and declared that cholesterol doesn't kill it sparked a war of words with a doctor who was one of my followers.

He claimed I was incorrect, misguiding people and declared that there was no evidence whatsoever to support my assertion. He demanded that I verify and provide evidence for my allegations.

That night I provided the research on my website along with video footage. Eventually, he went silent. I think it likely that he was in shock because he had never heard of or seen any such new research.

This is regrettable because the medical practice should keep up to date with what is happening in the field of medical research so that doctors can provide their patients with alternate treatments that could prove beneficial.

Things like this can cause future problems too. Not all doctors are going to be silent on the matter and others will not want to learn new things for the simple reason that they are too busy to attend to it.

 It's up to us ordinary folks to find our answers and seek out alternative methods of treatment that can be supported by research so that we don't accidentally embrace quack alternatives. We're the ones who are sick and have more to lose if we are not careful.

A word of caution; Placing your faith in one thing without keeping an open mind is like children believing in Santa Clause.
Even though the goal and intentions of the parents is noble, it doesn't mean that it's true.

There are many things in this world we can learn if we are daring enough to open our eyes and ears to discover, to listen but we should never silently accept things without question.

Open mindedness is a good thing, but don't be so open that you become like a waste basket where everything that is thrown at you is accepted.

Sometimes a case is made to look good but without clear empirical evidence.

Before I finish this book, I want to tickle you one more time.

Facts!!! How Good Having : Smoking

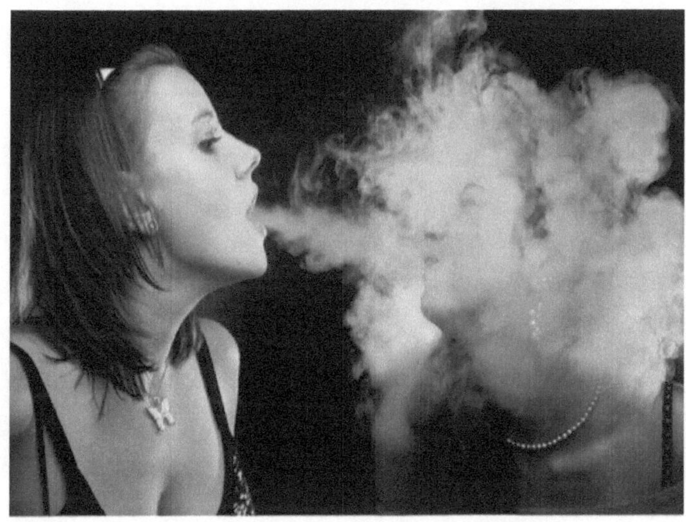

Passive Smoking Carries No Risk At All?

Did you know that there is recent research stating that Second Hand Smoke a.k.a passive smoking carries no risk at all? :)

The first time passive smoking was addressed and publicly identified as a health threat was in 1972. This led directly to the anti-smoking movement.

This issue wasaddressedagain in subsequent U.S. Surgeon GeneralReport'sin 1979, 1982, and 1984.

A 1986 Surgeon General's Report concluded that passive smoking causes lung cancer. But it offered only weak epidemiological evidence to support the claim. In 1989 the Environment Protection Agency (EPA) was charged with further evaluating the evidence for effects on health.

In 1992 the EPA published a report, "Respiratory Health Effects of Passive Smoking," claiming that passive smoking is a serious public health problem. They alleged that passive smoking kills approximately 3,000 nonsmoking Americans each year from lung cancer.
This report has been used by the tobacco-control movement and government agencies, including public health departments, to justify this and put thousands of indoor smoking bans in public places.

However, the EPA's 1992 report was not supported by reliable scientific evidence.
The report has been largely discredited and, in 1998, was legally vacated by a US federal judge.

For its 1992 report, the EPA arbitrarily chose to equate passive smokers with active smokers. One of the assumptions was that because there is an association between active smoking and lung cancer, there also must be a similar association between passive smoking and lung cancer.

But the problem posed by passive smoking is entirely different from that of active smoking. A toxicological principle: "The dose makes the poison."

In a study it was argued that those who were not active smokers, when placed next to active smokers, their greatest exposure to inhaling second hand smoke was the equivalent of one cigarette per day (around 0.03%) or the equivalent to smoking around 10 cigarettes per year.

EPA Studies rejected

In November 1995 after a 20-month study, the Congressional Research Service released a detailed analysis of the EPA report that was highly critical of EPA's methods and conclusions. In 1998, in a devastating 92-page opinion, Federal Judge William Osteen vacated the EPA study, declaring it null and void.
 He found a culture of arrogance, deception, and cover-up at the agency.

In 2003 a definitive paper on passive smoking and lung cancer mortality was published in the British Medical Journal. It is the largest and most detailed study ever reported.

The authors studied more than 35,000 California never-smokers over a 39-year period and found no statistically significant association between exposure to passive smoking and lung cancer mortality.

Millions of dollars have been spent promoting belief this as a killer, and it has been proven it is not true. Unfortunately this is not disseminated because people are afraid to accept the truth.
Indeed, we have to admit that smoking in front of people who don't smoke is really disturbing because it would take away their right to smoke-free clean air.

Most tragically, all of the research and controversy wasted millions of dollars. Imagine how much good those millions would have done if it had been invested in finding the true cause of lung cancer in non smokers.

On a final note; nothing that I write here is forever. Research is always evolving, always changing and always new information is discovered. What I have presented here is merely the most recent and it hasn't become well known to the public.
This is why I write this.
Keep an open mind to new things.

MD Official Quick Guide

This is MD :

1. No breakfast (minimal 3-4 hours after waking up) the reason was explained in the eBook

2. Eat 8/6/4 hours a day (outside those hours only drink plain water or tea without sugar) with this you can raise your HGH level.

3. If you are accustomed to a 4 hour eating pattern please try a 24 hour fast/eat once a day at a maximum of 3 times a week.

4. Eat what you normally eat before you begin the MD program

5. Exercise with weight lifting not cardio, fat burning will be maximized after 2 days in a row of weight lifting if you are fasting.

6. Fasting over 16 hours/day increases your HGH hormone by 1300%-2000% which is beneficial for restoring all the functions in your body with maximum fat burning

Thank you...
Author